Children and HIV/AIDS

Children and HIV/AIDS

Editors
Gary Anderson
Constance Ryan
Susan Taylor-Brown
Myra White-Gray

Routledge
Taylor & Francis Group
LONDON AND NEW YORK

Originally published as a special issue of *Child Welfare*, vol. 77, no. 2, March/April 1998 © 1998 by the Child Welfare League of America, Inc.

First published 1999 by Transaction Publishers

2 Park Square, Milton Park, Abingdon, Oxfordshire, OXI4 4RN
711 Third Avenue, New York, NY 10017

Routledge is an imprint of the Taylor and Francis Group, an informa business

First issued in hardback 2017

Library of Congress Catalog Number: 98–29901

Library of Congress Cataloging-in-Publication Data

Children and HIV/AIDS / edited by Gary Anderson . . . [et al.].
p. cm.
ISBN 0-7658-0488-3 (alk. paper)
1. Children of AIDS patients—Social aspects. 2. AIDS (Disease)—Patients—Family relationships. 3. AIDS (Disease) in children—Patients—Family relationships. 4. AIDS (Disease) in children—Patients—Services for. 5. AIDS (Disease) in children—Social aspects. I. Anderson, Gary R., 1952– .
RA644.A25C4479 1999
362.1'98929792—dc21 98-29901
CIP

ISBN 13: 978-0-7658-0488-4 (pbk)
ISBN 13: 978-1-138-52038-7 (hbk)

Contents

HIV AND ADOLESCENTS

Preface

HIV/AIDS and Children, Youths, and Families: Lessons Learned is a special issue of *Child Welfare* intended as a resource to personnel within the child welfare field serving children and families whose lives are touched by HIV and AIDS. It is our hope that this special issue will add insight to and fuel discussion of the fight against AIDS, and help us all to better serve the children and adolescents that the current epidemic affects so tragically.

Early in the AIDS epidemic, the Child Welfare League of America (CWLA) recognized that the disease would have a devastating impact on children, adolescents, and families. In response, CWLA established a National Task Force on Children and HIV Infection. Since June 1986, the Task Force has provided leadership and compassionate guidance to CWLA, its staff, and its member agencies from across the country on policy issues, program designs, and best practices concerning children and families living with HIV/AIDS. The task force was recently renamed the National Task Force on HIV Infection in Children, Adolescents, and Families to better reflect two major concerns: (1) that the heterosexual spread of AIDS among adolescents calls for continued emphasis on this often forgotten population, and (2) that the whole family of a child or parent infected with the virus must be perceived as the focus of community support and help.

Since its inception, the Task Force's leadership and guidance have expanded to encompass all community-based services for families, including child day care, out-of-home care, and group residential care programs that serve children with HIV. In 1987, CWLA published *Initial Guidelines on HIV Infection* to help child and family-serving agencies develop responsive and updated policies and procedures. Between 1989 and 1991, additional publications continued to further assist these programs.

In 1989, responding to the need for training and support for permanency planning recruitment of foster and adoptive families for children living with AIDS, CWLA produced an award-winning video, *With Loving Arms,* that has been used successfully throughout the country. CWLA's awareness that HIV prevention and education are the key to serving children, adolescents, and their families led it to offer information and services that have been used by thousands of social service agencies nationwide. These include the creation of the *Hugs InVited* training series (a joint project of CWLA and the Children's Hospital/Children's National Medical Center), the publication of several books, and the provision of direct training.

From 1991 to 1995, the number of women diagnosed with AIDS increased 63%, vastly increasing the number of children who will be affected by their mother's illness. In 1992, under the leadership of the Task Force's Subcommittee to Place Children Who Lose Their Parents to AIDS, CWLA designed a comprehensive initiative to support communities and service organizations that serve children affected by HIV/AIDS. The initiative has included policy guidelines, cross-systems training seminars, and resources for parents, children, professionals, volunteers, and public and private agencies.

This special issue of *Child Welfare* is another step forward in our ongoing fight against HIV/AIDS, and in our efforts to help those affected by it. The Task Force expresses its thanks to Gary Anderson, Professor, School of Social Work, Hunter College, New York, New York; Constance Ryan, Consultant, New Hope, Pennsylvania; Susan Taylor-Brown, Associate Professor, School of Social Work, Syracuse University, Syracuse, New York; and Myra White-Gray, FaCT Project Director, Maryland Department of Human Resources, Baltimore, Maryland, who helped make this issue possible by serving as its editors, and to all those who have contributed to this issue.

Despite recent medical advances, there is still no cure for HIV or AIDS. Combinations of new drugs and new knowledge are enabling persons with HIV to live much longer, however, they are also raising new issues for service providers trying to assist these persons and their families. We welcome your comments and reactions to this special issue and challenge all who work with children, youths, and their families to respond with creativity and innovation to the epidemic in your communities and nationwide.

DONNA PRESSMA
Chair, CWLA National Task Force on HIV Infection in Children, Adolescents, and Families

BRUCE HERSHFIELD
Director, CWLA HIV/AIDS Initiatives

INTRODUCTION

In December 1982, the Centers for Disease Control (CDC) began receiving the first reports of cases of children with HIV/AIDS. Since that time, the child welfare system, as well as other human service organizations, have been coping with and responding to the crises of children and families living with HIV/AIDS, including the considerable number of children affected by AIDS through the illness of their parents, siblings, or other family members.

Unfortunately, children who are not themselves infected with HIV frequently remain outside of the HIV service delivery network. Although not directly infected, these children are profoundly affected, as HIV disease can permanently alter their family structure. The HIV pandemic has had (and continues to have) a devastating impact on families. For example, following parental death, siblings are not always able to remain together.

Most of the children affected by HIV have been in the epicenters. Currently, however, communities outside of the HIV epicenters (also known as second-wave cities) are being confronted with increasing numbers of HIV-affected children and youths. Reflecting on the early experiences of the epicenters and building on their existing knowledge can assist the communities that are newly or increasingly being affected. Lessons have been learned that can be of benefit in the development and delivery of services, not only to HIV-affected children and families but to other families as well.

Lessons Learned

Extended Families Want to Care for Their Own

Initially, there was an impression that these young children had no families—their mothers were very ill, dying, or had abandoned the children. Their fathers were unknown, thought dead, or in prison. Extended family members were described as being afraid of AIDS, incompetent to care for children with HIV/AIDS, or were not identified. They were not seen as viable resources.

Experience has demonstrated that extended family members, godparents, and friends are stepping forward to care for affected children, and make up the majority of care providers today. Initially (and currently in too many areas), more resources were available to nonrelatives providing care (such as foster parents) than to relatives. The extension of similar resources to biological families has enabled many parents and relatives to care for or maintain an active role in their children's lives. Resources continue to be needed, however, to help keep siblings together in "second families."

Family Placements are Preferable to Group Homes or Institutions

In the early years of the HIV/AIDS epidemic, it was believed that it would be impossible to find anyone to care for children with HIV/AIDS, and some even advocated for the opening of group homes or institutions for these infants and children. Experience has demonstrated, however, that with careful and extensive recruiting, training, and support, relatives, foster parents, adoptive parents, and other caregivers have been successfully enlisted to care for these children.

Secrecy Exacerbates Stigma and Isolation

Confidentiality has been an ongoing concern—the prevailing belief was that children with HIV/AIDS should be kept apart from others and encouraged to maintain a strict secrecy about their illness, due to the stigma and discrimination associated with HIV.

The stigma associated with HIV/AIDS continues to be powerful, pervasive, and difficult to eliminate or reduce. Children, however, can and should be encouraged to live as full a life as possible in their communities. Total secrecy is being reevaluated, and perhaps modified so that children and young people can be more open about HIV. Disclosure of HIV status opens persons up to support and to opportunities to honestly express themselves.

The Needs of Adolescents Must Not Be Overlooked

The initial focus for child welfare was on infants and young children who acquired HIV/AIDS from their mothers. Because of the time that it takes to medically reach the criteria necessary for a definition of AIDS, the number of adolescents reported to the CDC has always been relatively low. The high number of AIDS cases among people in their 20s, however, makes it apparent that their infection with HIV happened during adolescence.

Throughout the epidemic, it has been a challenge to confront teen HIV infection. A public discomfort with addressing adolescents' sexual behaviors and drug use has contributed to this challenge. Prevention has always posed a formidable task, especially with an age group that feels relatively invulnerable and engages in risky behaviors. Educating and intervening with vulnerable teenagers in the community and in foster care, group homes, and residential treatment has been a needed focus throughout the AIDS crisis in the United States. Affected adolescents are particularly vulnerable and should be targeted for preventive efforts.

Focus on Living with HIV, Not Dying from HIV

In the early days of AIDS, there was often an attitude that children would die soon and that caregivers should therefore try to make their short lives as comfortable and happy as possible. Workers had to be trained to deal with death and dying and the foster home situation was similar to a hospice experience.

Today, due to a number of increasingly effective medications and supportive care, a great many children find they are living with HIV/AIDS, and are not awaiting impending death. Caregivers must nurture children's growth and development as the children mature, and must advocate for needed services.

HIV Affects the Total Family

As the number of persons infected by HIV continues to expand, so too does the number of children affected by the disease, although not themselves infected. Although the early focus was on children with HIV and AIDS, the focus has now expanded to encompass the large number of children who are affected by HIV/AIDS due to the diagnosis of their parents, relatives, or other caregivers and friends. Services must respond to the total family unit, not just the infected member.

Service Provision Must Be Culturally Sensitive and Competent

As is true of other aspects of the child welfare system, persons of color are overrepresented in the ranks of persons with HIV/AIDS. As of December 1996, the CDC reported that 31% of men with AIDS are African American, and 17% are Latino. Over 55% of the women with AIDS are African American, and over 20% are identified by the CDC as Latino.

Each racial and ethnic group has its own variety of beliefs about illness and disease, healing and medical care, and sexual behaviors and attitudes. Experiences and histories concerning the health care system and child welfare system in the United States are widely diverse. Services and research should therefore be culturally sensitive and based on thoughtful assessment and outreach.

Care Must Be Integrated and Comprehensive

Case management for children and youths with profound medical needs, as well as psychological, social, and spiritual needs, is challenging. A team of caregivers and professionals is needed to address not only the needs of the infected person, but of the whole family. Respite care for family and caregivers should be made available, and special supports put in place for sometimes medically fragile infants and children.

Permanency Planning Must Be Flexible

Permanency planning, a central policy and strategy for child welfare service delivery, took on new meaning as lessons were learned about the needs of children affected by HIV/AIDS, as well as concern for the long-term care of children whose parents were very ill and/or dying of AIDS. The need for early permanency planning—talking with parents about custodial and other issues for the care of their children—became an integral part of community services and foster care services for families.

Helping parents throughout the permanency planning process continues to be a major challenge. Permanency planning must remain a priority, but it must be recognized that creating such plans is an emotionally taxing experience for a parent and that plans change over time. To designate a guardian for one's children is to contemplate one's own death. Many parents, whether HIV-infected or not, are unable to do this. Service providers must foster the parent-child relationship, help parents with future planning, and be prepared to step in at the time of parental incapacity or death to ensure that the surviving children are kept together in a loving and caring environment. Too often, siblings are separated at the time of parental death. This complex situation has necessitated the addition of new members to the team of helping persons, such as lawyers, and posed continuing challenges in the development of multidisciplinary perspectives and teamwork to assist families. Foster parents in early permanency planning programs have become special resources to family members, frequently providing respite care in addition to out-of-home caregiving.

About This Book

This volume examines lessons learned from a variety of perspectives and settings, and identifies a number of continuing challenges facing the field. Although promising medications seem to encourage some optimism in the treatment of HIV/AIDS, the growing number and proportion of women with AIDS and the continuing rise of cases among persons of color sadly assure that more lessons will yet be learned from the AIDS crisis. We hope that what we have learned so far will improve the delivery of services for families affected by HIV, and will be generalizable to other challenges facing the child welfare system.

GARY ANDERSON
Professor, School of Social Work
Hunter College
New York, NY

CONSTANCE RYAN
Consultant
New Hope, PA

SUSAN TAYLOR-BROWN
Associate Professor,
School of Social Work
Syracuse University,
Syracuse, NY

MYRA WHITE-GRAY
FaCT Project Director
Maryland Department
of Human Resources
Baltimore, MD

1 HIV Infection and Children: A Medical Overview

A decade has passed since the Child Welfare League of America (CWLA) National Task Force on Children and HIV Infection published its *Initial Guidelines on HIV Infection*, a monograph that evolved in response to questions raised at a seminar sponsored by CWLA the previous year. At that 1987 seminar, "Attention to AIDS," a compelling need to develop sound child welfare policy based on incomplete but best available medical experience was voiced, and CWLA took the lead in responding. Ten years later, despite multiple advances in medical care, the social, medical, and legal challenges of HIV/AIDS continue to affect children, families, and communities. The need to promote best practice through training, research, and literature remains paramount.

HIV Transmission

The medical overview I wrote in 1988 for CWLA's *Initial Guidelines* focused on HIV transmission. There was a clear need to counter the epidemic of fear and prejudice associated with HIV with knowledge of how HIV is and is not transmitted. Fortunately, clinical experience and time have confirmed that HIV is not transmitted by casual contact and that the risk to health care providers and child care workers is remote if universal precautions are observed. HIV does not spread in households through activities of daily living or hugging an infected person. Although HIV can be transmitted through exposure to infected blood or body secretions, universal precautions—the use of latex gloves and bleach when contact must be made with those fluids—can prevent transmission. HIV proliferates in white blood cells; thus, infected blood must be in direct contact with the blood of an uninfected person through a break in the skin or mucous membranes for a new HIV infection to occur. The odds of exposure to bodily secretions and blood is greatest during anal receptive intercourse, the sharing of intravenous drug paraphernalia with an infected person, and vaginal heterosexual intercourse. Prior to the development of the HIV antibody test in 1985, HIV-contaminated blood products were a major source of HIV infection, especially to those dependent on those products, such as hemophiliacs. The nation's blood supply is now tested routinely for HIV, and the risk of acquiring HIV through a blood transfusion is extremely remote.

HIV can also be transmitted from an infected mother to her child, either prenatally or during childbirth. Most infantile HIV is acquired during delivery; infection in the womb or via breast feeding accounts for only about 10% of infant HIV cases in the United States. When transmission of HIV to the infant occurred can now be determined through testing at or during the first few weeks following birth. A positive viral culture or polymerase chain reaction (PCR) assay for HIV at birth indicates intrauterine HIV transmission. HIV can destroy the immune systems of infants infected in utero before such systems have a chance to develop. These infants have high viral loads and tend to get sick in early infancy. Infants who are viral culture and PCR negative at birth but test positive after seven days have likely acquired HIV by swallowing infected maternal blood or cervical secretions during birth. These infants have a lower viral load and remain asymptomatic for a longer time than those infected in utero.

Diagnosis and Treatment of HIV in Infants

Early awareness of infant HIV status is extremely important. It affects not only the child's potential placement for adoption or out-of-home care, but also the course of treatment undertaken. Until recently, the presence of maternal HIV antibodies in an infant's blood made early diagnosis of the infant's own HIV status nearly impossible. Typically, 15 months had to elapse before a child free of symptoms could be declare to be free of HIV. Advances in testing now allow early establishment of an infant's HIV status—the results of three viral cultures or PCRs during the first month of life can prove or rule out HIV infection. The ability to identify HIV-infected infants at or near birth has made possible the early treatment of HIV-positive children, and improved assessment of the effectiveness of treatment.

New drugs and combinations of drugs allow therapy to be tailored to individual needs. In 1988, the only drug available to treat HIV was AZT. Today, analogues such as 3TC or DDI are available if toxicity or resistance to AZT develops. Positive clinical responses to protease inhibitors are also raising new hope. Difficulties in the use of these drugs in children must still be overcome, however. Most have not been officially approved for use in children, although anecdotal evidence supports high expectations for clinical improvement. Some of the drugs taste bad, are not available in liquid form, have prohibitive costs, promote resistant strains of HIV if compliance is poor, or may lead to other medical problems such as diabetes. The introduction of new classes of drugs is exciting, but only time can determine the risk-benefit ratio of each.

HIV destroys the immune system by infecting CD4+T helper cells. Monitoring levels of CD4 cells in the peripheral blood allows treatment providers to chart the progression of HIV disease and to recognize an increased risk for opportunistic infection. Improved therapy for these infections are prolonging the lives of HIV-infected children. For example, in 1988, 60% of children with AIDS died from pneumocystis carinii pneumonia (PCP), an opportunistic infection. Today, a low T cell count can indicate when Bactrim prophylaxis for PCP should be prescribed, and death from PCP has become a rare event. Improved therapies for other opportunistic infections, especially cytomegalovirus, fungal infections, and tuberculosis, and timely use of childhood vaccination as well as the antipneumococcal vaccine, are helping to prevent complicating infections in immune-deficient children.

Maternal Treatment and Testing

At present, pediatric AIDS accounts for less than 2% of the total number of AIDS cases in the United States. Ninety percent of these children acquired their infection at birth. In 1988, 25% to 50% of infants born to HIV-positive mothers acquired the infection. With changes in maternal and newborn treatment, that number has dropped to 6% to 8%.

Most HIV-positive pregnant women today do not have AIDS but are in a relatively asymptomatic phase of infection. They may discover their infection only during routine prenatal care, where they are counseled to have an HIV test. HIV-positive pregnant women are typically referred to special programs where AZT during pregnancy, labor, and delivery is offered as a standard of care, in accord with federal recommendations; their newborn children are also given AZT as a prophylactic. In 1994, AZT administration to HIV-infected pregnant women helped reduce maternal fetal HIV transmission by 67% in the United States.

Competing concerns have thwarted sensible public health law since the onset of the epidemic. In some states, HIV testing of pregnant women is mandatory, a practice that has resulted in a political and social firestorm. Opponents of mandatory testing argue that, although it may help prevent some cases of pediatric AIDS, it violates a women's autonomy if she would rather not be tested.

Similarly, the routine testing of newborns for HIV has raised a controversy. For example, in New York State, tests were performed on the umbilical cord blood of all newborns for more than 12 years, although mothers were not routinely informed of the results. Epidemiologists used this information to track the burden of HIV in various communities. Starting in March 1997, all new mothers began receiving the results of their infants' umbilical cord tests. A positive test on the infant's blood indicates that the mother has HIV. This information can be a grave shock to a new mother; it also raises strong feelings of guilt since the mother receives this information too late to receive AZT and protect her child. While the New York State policy was established in part due to a high resistance to prenatal maternal testing, critics argue that it demonstrates a blatant disregard for both the mother's free choice and the newborn's best interest.

Advances and Challenges

In the past few years, several significant medical advances have changed the face of the HIV/AIDS epidemic.

- AZT, administered during pregnancy and parturition, has dramatically reduced the rate of maternal-infant transmission.
- Highly sensitive and specific molecular genetic PCR assays have proven themselves to be as accurate as a viral cultures in determining HIV infection, making it possible to identify HIV-infected newborns in the first month of life.
- Protease inhibitors and other new treatments for HIV are being developed and refined.
- Viral load studies are being used to closely monitor the effectiveness of antiretroviral treatment.
- The measurement of CD4+T helper cells is being used to track HIV's progression in individuals, leading to a reduction in and prompt treatment of bacterial and opportunistic infections.
- Side effects of infection and treatment are being better controlled, with improved strategies for pain management.
- Growth factors such as Epogen are now used to support bone marrow functioning and prevent anemia.
- Increased attention is being focused on the nutritional needs of HIV-infected individuals.

Although increased knowledge of HIV has lessened the fear associated with it and increased society's tolerance, many challenges remain.

- As new medical treatments evolve for HIV, we run the risk of becoming complacent. The search must continue for an HIV vaccine to protect the uninfected and stop viral replication in those already HIV infected. New drugs must be tested in pediatric clinical trials and formulated for use in children. Procedures should be established for garnering "fast track" approval of promising treatments for compassionate use. Quality health care that is accessible, affordable, and cost effective must be made available.

- The increasing incidence of unsafe sexual practices (especially the failure to use condoms properly) and the increase in the spread of sexually transmitted diseases other than HIV indicate a continuing need for education. High risk-taking behavior by youths must be discouraged. Schools must provide age-appropriate sexuality education. All medical and social welfare providers should receive continuing AIDS awareness education and should promote AIDS awareness and prevention in all clinical encounters. Continuing education should be provided for caregivers, families, and the general public as new information becomes available. HIV infected persons need to know their serostatus and protect their sexual partners.
- The need to reach out in a culturally appropriate manner to gay youths and to minority women and teenagers remains strong. We must empower women, minorities, teenagers, and other vulnerable persons who are not able to negotiate sexual activity. The transmission of HIV through rape and child sexual abuse must be ended.

Conclusion

By definition, an epidemic is not confined to a single segment of the population; likewise, its impact is not limited to public health, but encompasses a broad range of social issues. A child never has HIV in isolation. Often, an infected father transmits the disease to his sexual partner, who then passes HIV on to her infant. The range of challenges requires a mesh of the expertise of both medical and social workers. Multidisciplinary, family-oriented patient care review conferences on a regular basis can be used to evaluate the quality and effectiveness of team interventions. Coordination of services can result in cost savings and can provide an organized, cohesive method that prioritizes the families' needs in a holistic manner. Systems of care must prepare and assist service providers to assess needs, provide tangible and intangible supports, and to deal with death, dying, and bereavement. Ideally, we must integrate health services with social services and involve the whole family—those infected as well as those affected—for the social difficulties the HIV epidemic raises are just as challenging as the medical concerns.

VIRGINIA ANDERSON, M.D.
Director of Pediatric Pathology
SUNY Health Science Center, Brooklyn
Kings County Medical Center
Brooklyn, NY

Supporting References

Anderson, V. M. (1987). AIDS as it affects children and adolescents. In *Attention to AIDS: Proceedings of a seminar responding to the growing number of children and youth with AIDS.* Washington, DC: Child Welfare League of America.

Anderson, V. M. (1988). HIV infection and children: A medical overview. In D. Pressma & J. L. Emery (Eds.), *Initial Guidelines: Report of the CWLA Task Force on Children and HIV Infection*. Washington, DC: Child Welfare League of America.

Chervenak, F. A., & McCullough, L. B. (1996). Common ethical dilemmas encountered in the management of HIV-infected women and newborns. *Clinical Obstetrics and Gynecology*, 39, 411–9.

Beisel, W. R. (1996). Nutrition in pediatric HIV infection: Setting the research agenda. Nutrition and immune function overview. *Journal of Nutrition, 126*, 2611S–2615S.

Grubman, S., & Simonds, R. J. (1996). Preventing pneumocystis carinii pneumonia in human immunodeficiency virus-infected children: New guidelines for prophylaxis. Centers for Disease Control, U.S. Public Health Service and the Infectious Disease Society of America. *Pediatric Infectious Disease Journal, 15*,165–8.

Hirschfeld, S. (1996). Dysregulation of growth and development in HIV-infected children. *Journal of Nutrition, 126*, 2641S–2650S.

Lambert, J. S. (1996). Pediatric HIV infection. *Current Opinions in Pediatrics, 8*, 606–14.

Larson, T., & Bechtel, L. (1995). Managing the child infected with HIV. *Primary Care Clinics in Office Practice, 22*, 23–50.

Lewis, S. L., Wesley, Y., & Haiken, H. J. (1996). Pediatric and family HIV: Psychosocial concerns along the continuum of disease. *Nursing Clinicians of North America, 31,* 221–30.

Lindsay, M. K. (1996). Routine voluntary antepartum HIV antibody counseling and testing: A sound public health prevention strategy. *Clinical Obstetrics and Gynecology, 39,* 305–15.

Lindsay, M. K., & Nesheim, S. R. (1997). Human immunodeficiency virus infection in pregnant women and their newborns. *Clinical Perinatology 24,* 161–80.

McClain, K. L., Joshi, V. V., & Murphy, S. B. (1996). Cancers in children with HIV infection. *Hematology Oncology Clinics of North America 10,* 1189–201.

McKinney, R. E. Jr. (1996). Antiretroviral therapy: Evaluating the new era in HIV treatment. *Advances in Pediatric Infectious Disease 12,* 297–323.

Myhre, J. A., Chadwick, E. G., & Yogev, R. (1996). Failure to thrive in HIV-infected children: Incidence, prevalence and clinical correlates. *Pediatric AIDS and HIV Infection, 7,* 83–90.

Wilfert, C. M., Gross, P. A., Kaplan, J. E., Holmes, K. K., Masur, H., Phair, J. P., & Simonds, R. J. (1995). Quality standard for the enumeration of CD4+ lymphocytes in infants and children exposed to or infected with immunodeficiency virus. *Clinical Infectious Disease, 21,* S134–5.

Wu, L. R., Capparelli, E. V., & Connor, J. D. (1995). Therapy of pediatric AIDS. *Current Opinions in Pediatrics, 7,* 214–9.

2 Factors Associated with Parents' Decision to Disclose Their HIV Diagnosis to Their Children

Lori S. Wiener, Haven B. Battles, and Nancy E. Heilman

Parents report that trying to decide whether or not to disclose their HIV diagnosis to their children is as emotionally charged as learning of the diagnosis itself. As part of a larger study, interviews were conducted with 17 parent-child dyads recruited from patients being treated at the National Cancer Institute to understand the factors that affect the process of disclosure of a parent's HIV diagnosis and its consequences. Parents and HIV-infected children were also interviewed and were administered several standardized measures for collecting information on parental depression, family environment, and social support satisfaction. The factors associated with a parent's decision to disclose his or her diagnosis to the children, and implications for clinical practice and future research, are discussed.

Lori S. Wiener, Ph.D., ACSW, is Coordinator, Pediatric HIV Psychosocial Support Program; and Haven B. Battles, M.Phil., is Research Associate, HIV/AIDS Malignancy Branch, National Cancer Institute, Bethesda, MD. Nancy E. Heilman, Ph.D., is Child Psychologist, Good Samaritan Hospital, Puyallup, Washington.

I was hesitant to share the diagnosis with others. I was afraid that people would reject me or my child. Disclosure was a big struggle...about how, when, and what I would do. But it didn't turn out as bad as I thought it would.

—*HIV-infected mother of three*

AIDS is the leading cause of death among adults age 25 to 44 in the United States [Centers for Disease Control 1996b]. As of December 1996, 85,500 women of childbearing age (13 to 44) were reported as having AIDS [Centers for Disease Control 1996a]. Many of these women have young children to whom they must, at some point, consider disclosing their diagnosis. This is a stressful decision to make, not only because of the fatal nature of the disease, but because disclosing an HIV diagnosis often entails a conversation about parental acquisition of the virus. In addition, disclosing the parents' diagnosis may lead to a disclosure of the child's diagnosis, if the child is HIV-infected as well.

Several studies have examined a person's decision to disclose his or her HIV diagnosis to others. Derlega et al. [in press] found that among adults with HIV, the primary reasons for disclosing to significant others were (in descending order of frequency): (1) a desire for emotional closeness with, or support from, others; (2) a forewarning to significant others; (3) health/transmission concerns; (4) a desire to be honest with others; (5) a need for tangible assistance (e.g., informational material); (6) situational factors (e.g., friend accompanied them to get test results); (7) a desire to educate others; (8) feelings of loyalty to significant others; (9) ease of disclosure to someone with a similar background; (10) catharsis or self-expression; and (11) testing of others' reactions. Reasons for nondisclosure included: (1) a fear of rejection or ostracism; (2) a desire to protect the feelings of significant others; (3) a fear that others would gossip; (4) a fear of ignorance; (5) uncertainty about how to disclose; (6) a desire to keep others from making sacrifices; or (7) geographic separation (e.g., did not want to disclose over the telephone).

Although they did not ask reasons for disclosure, Hays et al. [1993] cited reasons for nondisclosure among their sample of HIV-positive gay men: (1) not wanting to worry or upset others; (2) fear of discrimination; (3) fear of disrupting relationships; (4) emotional self-protection; (5) feeling that the other person would have little to offer that would be beneficial; (6) feeling a lack of intimacy with the other individual; and (7) a desire to conceal one's homosexuality. Many of the reasons to disclose revolved around the desire to improve on or maintain a close relationship with significant others. Likewise, reasons for nondisclosure often included a desire to protect or avoid negative feedback from significant others. These are all factors thought to be relevant to the question of disclosure within a parent-child relationship.

Few studies have examined the factors associated with disclosure of parental HIV to a child. Pliskin et al. [1993] found that 55% of their sample of HIV-infected mothers disclosed their diagnosis to their non-HIV-infected children; the remainder did not. The mothers who did disclose expressed one or more of the following reasons for doing so: (1) an opposition to family secrets; (2) a wish to psychologically prepare their children; (3) a desire for greater intimacy with their children; and (4) a wish to prevent their children from learning the diagnosis from someone outside the family. Mothers who did not disclose their diagnosis reported one or more of the following reasons: (1) a fear that their children would be psychologically harmed (e.g., poor school performance, ostracism, excessive worry); (2) a desire to preserve their children's childhood; (3) a belief that their children lacked the intellectual capacity to understand the diagnosis; and (4) a fear that their children would reject them. These reasons for disclosure and nondisclosure are similar to those expressed by the men in the earlier studies.

The present study sought to assess the variables associated with the process of disclosure of a parent's HIV diagnosis to his or her child and its consequences. Results of previous research and clinical work formed the basis for an interview administered to the study participants. Parents were also asked a number of questions either about the disclosure experience, or about how they envisioned the disclosure experience if they had not yet disclosed.

Method

These data were collected as part of a larger study that examined three different components of disclosure. The first component described the parent's decision to disclose or not to disclose the child's HIV diagnosis to the child [Wiener et al. 1996]. The second component, which is reported here, examined factors associated with the parents' decision to disclose or not to disclose their own HIV diagnosis to their children. The third component examined the factors underlying public disclosure of a child's HIV diagnosis [Wiener et al. in press]. In the part of the study reported here, 17 families in which both the child and the parent were HIV-infected were interviewed. All of the children were patients being treated at the pediatric branch of the National Cancer Institute (NCI).

Participants

Children between the ages of five and 18 were eligible for the larger study. One hundred fifty parent-child dyads were identified for participation. Of these, 123 children had appointments during the time the study was being conducted and therefore were available to participate. Ninety-nine of these children were able to complete all of the measures, resulting in a response rate of 66%. Of those 99, 17 had caregivers who were HIV infected and thus were eligible for the parent disclosure arm of the study. All agreed to participate.

All of these caregivers were the children's biological parents. Of the 17 families interviewed, seven (41%) of the parents had disclosed their own diagnosis to their children and 10 (59%) had not. Eleven (65%) of the children were Caucasian, four (24%) were African American, and two (12%) were Latino. Ten (59%) were male, and seven (41%) were female. The mean age was 7.6 years. Of the parents, 16 (94%) were female and one (6%) was male. Two families had more than one HIV-infected child living in the household, two families had already lost one child to HIV, and nine families had one or more non-HIV-infected child(ren) in addition to their HIV-infected child in the household. In four families, the HIV-infected child was their only living child in the home.

Procedure

Parents were informed of the study by their social worker and were invited to participate. Appropriate referrals were made for any participants who disclosed information via questionnaire or interview that suggested that they were a danger to themselves or others, or that they otherwise required psychiatric intervention (e.g., met diagnostic criteria for depression or anxiety disorder).

The study's purpose was explained to parents and informed consent was obtained. Parents were asked to complete the Beck Depression Inventory (BDI) [Beck 1967] and the Family Environment Scale (FES) [Moos & Moos 1993]. Children between the ages of eight and 13 were administered the Self-Perception Profile for Children (SPPC) [Harter 1985] and children between the ages of 14 and 18 were administered the Harter Self-Perception Profile for Adolescents (SPPA) [Harter 1988].

Measures

Disclosure interview. This structured interview was designed by the investigators to elicit information on factors associated with the parent's decision to disclose or not to disclose HIV-related information to the child. The interview consisted of open-ended questions regarding the factors behind the parent's decision, including whether or not the health care team had any influence over the decision. For those who did disclose, the interview explored perceptions of how the child reacted to the disclosure, whether the parent's relationship with the child had changed since disclosure or since the original diagnosis, and whether the child seemed to have changed in general since learning his or her own diagnosis.

The Beck Depression Inventory [Beck 1967]. This 21-item, multiple-choice measure was completed by the primary parent to assess the frequency of symptoms of depression. Scores can range from 0 to 63; scores of 0 to 9 are in the normal range or asymptomatic, scores of 10 to 18 represent mild-moderate depression, scores of 19 to 29 are indicative of moderate-severe depression, and scores of 30 to 63 indicate extremely severe depression.

Arizona Social Support Interview Schedule [Barrera & Ainley 1983]. This scale measures the many facets of social support by obtaining quantitative information on positive and negative social contacts. This measure yields five social support indices: total network size, unconflicted network size, conflicted network size, support satisfaction, and support need. Only the last two indices were analyzed for this study. The *support satisfaction* subscale score is ascertained by asking, for each of the four unconflicted interactions, whether respondents would have liked (1) a lot more opportunities to...(e.g., talk to people about their personal and private feelings), (2) a few more opportunities, or (3) their support system was about right. *Support need* is determined by asking whether subjects felt they needed, for example, to talk about things that were very personal and private (1) not at all, (2) a little bit, or (3) quite a bit.

Family Environment Scale [Moos & Moos 1993]. This measure includes 10 subscales, with nine True/False items each. Subjects were administered the entire scale, but only two subscales are of interest for this analysis: the Cohesion scale, which assesses the degree of commitment, help, and support members provide for one another; and the Expressiveness scale, which assesses the extent to which members are encouraged to act openly and express feelings directly. High scores on cohesion and expressiveness are favorable; they do not represent families that are highly enmeshed in each other's lives or that are expressive to the point of excessive confrontation.

Self-Perception Profile for Children and Self-Perception Profile for Adolescents [Harter 1985, 1988]. These instruments measure the construct of self-perceived competence. The child form (ages eight to 13) consists of six subscales (scholastic, social, athletic, physical, behavioral, and global self-competence); the adolescent form contains nine (the six in the child form, plus romantic, job, and friend subscales).

Results

Parent Interview: Disclosers

All of the children in the disclosure group (*n*=7) were aware of both their parents' HIV diagnosis as well as their own. The average age for the children in this group was 9.3 years (ranging from six to 13 years), and the average length of time between diagnosis and disclosure was 2.5 years (ranging from two months to almost seven years). When asked the reasons for disclosing their own diagnosis to their child, two parents did not want their child to hear about the diagnosis from someone outside the family, two children found out accidentally, one parent wanted the child to be prepared for the mother's eventual death, one parent was opposed to family secrets, and one child asked specifically if they (mother and daughter) had AIDS. When asked why they disclosed at the time when they did, most of the reasons related primarily to the disclosure of the child's diagnosis and secondarily to the disclosure of the parents'. Two parents reported that their child was starting a protocol at NCI and they felt that was an appropriate time to disclose, two children asked specific questions about AIDS, two parents were concerned about possible transmission of the virus from their child to others (and so a disclosure of the child's diagnosis entailed a disclosure of their own), and one parent did not have a specific reason. Four of the parents had also told their other children (those not being seen at NCI for HIV infection) about their own diagnosis, two had not told their other children and one had no other children. Those who told their other children first generally did so because their other children were older and judged by the parent as better able to understand the diagnosis.

Parents were also asked what were their greatest concerns about disclosure before it took place. Two parents feared that their children would focus on death and/or give up on life, two parents feared that their children would be ostracized by others, one parent was afraid that her child would tell others about the diagnoses, one parent did not want her child to hate her, and one parent feared that the child would not be able to handle the information emotionally.

Parents were asked how their lives had changed since disclosing to their children. Parents of three children indicated that their lives had changed for the worse (i.e., one parent found herself becoming more withdrawn, another felt less accepted by others), two indicated no change, and two said their lives had changed for the better (i.e., life had become more calm). The parents were also asked how their relationship with their children had changed since disclosure. Five indicated no change, two indicated a positive change (i.e., family became closer), and none said their relationships had worsened. When asked if they would have changed the timing of their disclosure, all said they either would have done it at the same time (five) or sooner (two).

When asked how their children reacted to learning the diagnoses (of both parent and child), three said their children started asking questions, two said their children were scared, and two reported that their children had no reaction. Parents were asked what changes they had seen in their children since disclosure. Three reported no change, two reported change for the better, and two reported change for the worse. When parents were asked how they felt immediately after disclosure, four reported feeling relieved. Parents reported that disclosing was "a relief. It was a weight off my shoulders. I felt more in control," and "It was a relief, because I had been pushing it (not telling) for a while." Two parents reported feeling overwhelmed and one felt nervous.

Six of the parents reported that the NCI health care team positively affected their decision to disclose, while one reported a negative effect. When asked how often they thought about whether or not to disclose the diagnosis prior to disclosure, two parents reported thinking about it once a day, three reported a few times per week, and one reported a few times per month or less. When asked to what extent they struggled with the problem, four reported struggling tremendously, one reported struggling a little, and one reported struggling hardly at all (one parent was not asked the last two questions as she was added after the first few interviews were completed).

Parent Interview: Nondisclosers

All of the children in this group (n=10) were unaware of both their parents' and their own HIV diagnoses. The child's average age in this group was 6.5 years (ranging from 5 to 10 years). When the nondisclosing parents were asked their reasons for not disclosing their own diagnosis to their child, four thought their child would be psychologically harmed by the information. Reflecting this fear, one father said: "Children who know [their diagnosis] lack a spark in their eyes and the burden is something that they don't need as a tender child. My son is unencumbered by all of this emotional stuff and he is happy with that." Three parents felt their children lacked the intellectual capacity to understand the diagnosis, two wanted to preserve the innocence of childhood, and one feared her child would reject her. When asked if they had plans to disclose their diagnosis to their children, six indicated that they did and four didn't. Likewise, two parents planned to tell their non-HIV-infected children of their diagnosis, two had already told their other children, two did not plan to tell the other children, and four had no other children.

Parents were asked what factors would have to be in place before they would consider disclosing the diagnosis to the child. Seven parents indicated that they would tell their children when they were old enough to understand the diagnosis, one said she would tell if the child asked, one was waiting for the "right time," and one said she would never tell.

Parents were asked how they expected their children to react when they were informed of the parents' diagnosis. Four felt their children would be sad or worried, two thought they would be scared, two thought they would be accepting, one thought her child probably already knew, and one didn't know how her child would react. When asked what they would do if the child came out and asked if they had HIV or AIDS, seven indicated that they would tell the truth and three said they would still keep the information from the child.

Nine of the parents said that the health care team at NCI had no bearing on their decision not to disclose, while one indicated that the team had a negative effect (the team members were trying to persuade her to disclose, but she wouldn't). Four parents indicated that this was an issue they thought about at least once per day, one thought about it a few times per week, three thought about it once per week, and two thought about it a few times per month or less.

Psychosocial Variables

Since there were relatively few people in this sample, nonparametric tests were used to analyze the data. Means and standard deviations for the two groups on the standardized measures are presented in table 1. Using the nonparametric Wilcoxon 2-group test to test for differences in the means between the two groups (and using a critical values table for small sample sizes [Ott 1993; Wilcoxon & Wilcox 1964]), nondisclosers scored significantly higher on the Beck Depression Inventory (BDI) than did disclosers, ($z = -1.57, p = .12$). On the one hand, 57% of disclosers scored in the normal range for depression, and 43% scored in the mild to moderate range. On the other hand, 30% of nondisclosers scored in the normal range, 40% in the mild to moderate range, 20% in the moderate to severe range, and 10% in the extremely severe range. Disclosers' scored 8.1 out of 9 on the Cohesion and 6.6 out of 9 on the Expressiveness subscales of the Family Environment Scale (FES), while the nondisclosers scored 5.7 and 5.1, respectively. The mean Cohesion score for normal and distressed families, based on normative samples, are 6.61

TABLE 1
Means and Standard Deviations of Parental Disclosers and Nondisclosers on Depression, Family Environment, Social Support, and Child's Perceived Self-Competence

Measure	*Disclosers (n=7)*		*Nondisclosers (n=10)*	
	Mean	*SD*	*Mean*	*SD*
Beck Depression Inventory	8.3	6.5	15.5	11.3
Family Environment—Cohesion	8.1	1.2	5.7	3.1
Family Environment—Expressiveness	6.6	1.7	5.1	2.4
Social Support Need	2.1	0.4	2.2	0.5
Social Support Satisfaction	2.5	0.2	2.3	0.8
Child's perceived self-competence—scholastic	3.1	0.7	3.3	0.6
Child's perceived self-competence—social	2.8	0.9	2.6	0.2
Child's perceived self-competence—athletic	3.0	0.8	3.7	0.3
Child's perceived self-competence—physical	3.0	0.4	3.1	0.4
Child's perceived self-competence—behavioral	3.3	0.5	3.4	0.1
Child's perceived global self-competence	3.5	0.5	3.6	0.3

and 5.03, respectively, and 5.45 and 4.60 for Expressiveness [Moos & Moos 1993]. There was a significant difference ($z = 1.75$, $p = .08$) between disclosers and nondisclosers on the Cohesion subscale of the FES, with disclosers being more cohesive than nondisclosers. There were no significant differences between the two groups for the Expressiveness subscale of the FES, need for social support or satisfaction, or for the child's perceived self-competence.

Discussion

Clearly, one of the most difficult questions that parents struggle with after learning that they are HIV positive is whether or not to share this information with their dependent children. Although the majority of parents in this study indicated thinking about disclosure frequently (at least once a week), resistance to disclosure is common. Years may go by before the parent feels the time is appropriate to communicate this reality. Fifty-nine percent of the sample of parents had not yet disclosed their diagnosis to their children.

The emotional toll of concealing the diagnosis cannot be minimized. The finding that nondisclosing parents were more depressed than disclosing parents coincided with the findings from the larger study [Wiener et al. 1996], where parents who had disclosed the child's diagnosis to the child were significantly less depressed than those who had not disclosed. The stress of keeping a secret from one's own child—particularly a secret of this magnitude and relevance, and especially in households where one child has been informed of the parent's diagnosis and the other children are asked to keep silent about it—may well contribute to depressive symptoms. Alternatively, however, depressed parents may not have the psychological resources to communicate with their children and explain their illness honestly. The direction of this relationship is not clear. Further attention to depression in parents of HIV-infected children is warranted.

Nondisclosers' beliefs about how their children would react if told the diagnosis echoed their concern about disclosure in the first place. Most felt that their children would be sad or scared, while only a couple felt that their children would be accepting of the information. This coincides with the actual reactions of the children who were told. The majority appeared sad or concerned (asking questions), while two seemed to have no visible reaction to it at all. After sharing the diagnosis, some parents reported feeling so relieved that "it was over" that they described not having the emotional energy to talk about it again for some time. It is often not until days or weeks after disclosure takes place that the child has the courage to ask more questions. Therefore, before proceeding with disclosure, it is important for disclosing parents to identify a supportive adult who will be available to help the children process and cope with the information given.

For those who had disclosed, their greatest concern about disclosure (before doing so) was fear that their children would be harmed in some way (either due to the emotional impact of the information or to ostracism from others). For those who had not disclosed, their reasons primarily reflected their belief that their child was not intellectually capable of understanding the diagnosis or their desire to shield a young child from potentially harmful information. The concerns about disclosure and the reasons for not disclosing expressed in this study echoed the themes that emerged in the Pliskin et al. [1993] study, namely, that the children would be psychologically harmed, that they would lose the innocence of childhood, that they were not old or mature enough to understand the diagnosis, or that they would reject the parent.

Clinical observations have shown that discussion of a parent's HIV diagnosis often leads to other disclosures, many of which have previously remained family secrets. Some of these include a biological parent's true identity, the identity of others in the family who have AIDS or who have died of the disease, and the manner in which the disease was transmitted [Lipson 1994]. Due to fear of rejection, mothers in particular, who are struggling with guilt that their behavior or personal choices caused the disease, are often the most resistant to disclosing the diagnosis. The longer they had withheld the diagnosis, the more embedded the lies became and the harder it became to disclose. Parents often fear that their child will no longer trust them. Children frequently feel embarrassed that other people in their family have been aware of the diagnosis before they had been informed. Once disclosure takes place, these issues and feelings can be successfully dealt with in individual and conjoint counseling sessions with the parents and children.

The average age of the children in the disclosure group was 9.3 years, whereas the average age in the nondisclosure group was 6.5. Seven of the 10 parents who had not disclosed said they would do so when the child was old enough to understand the diagnosis.

Many parents are hesitant to disclose the diagnosis of a terminal illness to their child (their own or someone else's) because they feel the child is too young to understand the implications. While this may be true for very young children (under the age of two), research has demonstrated that children have at least a rudimentary understanding of death at around age three [Stambrook & Parker 1987]. Between the ages of three and five, children realize that death occurs. They may view death, however, as reversible and as happening only to other people. Rather than viewing death as a cessation of all life functions, they tend to think that the dead retain at least some of their capacities [Stambrook & Parker 1987; Sigelman & Shaffer 1995]. They often fear separation from loved ones more than they fear actual death. Between the ages of 6 and 10, children tend to realize that death is final and universal and they may begin to develop personal fears about it [Grollman 1995; Husband 1984; Pennells & Smith 1995]. Deasy-Spinetta [1981] has suggested that it is useless to attempt to shield children from the knowledge that they have a serious or terminal illness once they have reached this developmental stage. Based on the results of this study, it appears that parents are able to sense this readiness in their children when they reach this stage. Likewise, the larger study found that by age 11, 98% of the children in the sample had been told of their own diagnosis [Wiener et al. 1996].

This is not to say that everyone plans to disclose their diagnosis. Four of the 10 nondisclosers did not have specific plans to tell their child (although three thought that they would eventually), and one of them claimed that she would never tell her child, no matter what. Seven of these parents thought that if their child asked them directly about the diagnosis, they would then tell the truth.

While disclosers did not indicate an overwhelming feeling of positive change since disclosure, none said their relationships with their children had worsened. Of some concern, however,was the report by about one-third of the respondents who said their lives had worsened since they disclosed their diagnosis to their children. Clinical observations tell us that in these cases, prior to disclosure, the parents were able to "stay in denial" about the disease. Once the children were informed, the parents felt that they could no longer protect them emotionally from the painful reality of what the future could bring, especially when the children wanted to talk frequently about the disease. As one parent reported, "It has become emotionally exhausting to have to live with this disease not only in my mind but with my children now too." Interestingly, all of the parents in this study said that if they had to do it over, they would have done it at the same time or sooner. Thus, while the decision to disclose is obviously a difficult one, parents who have shared their diagnosis with their children are unanimous in their belief that it was the right decision.

Both groups reported nearly identical feelings about how the health care team at NCI had affected their decision to disclose or not to disclose. For the disclosers, six out of seven felt that the team had a positive impact on their decision, as did nine out of the 10 nondisclosers. One mother who had disclosed to her son said "[My social worker] had the biggest impact. She explained reasons for lying, and for being honest. I decided it would be better to be honest." Another mother reported that talking with her health care team helped her to feel "confident enough to tell my daughter [the diagnosis]. They didn't push or pressure me to do it." Only one in each group felt that the team had a negative impact on the decision (or was not supportive of the parents' chosen process of disclosure).

Talking to children about a parent's HIV disease takes preparation. The team can help prepare the parent, role-play possible scenarios, be with the parent at the time of disclosure if that is her or his wish, and be available to the parent and child following disclosure for additional support. It is important, however, that the parents not feel coerced into sharing their diagnosis with their children before they are adequately prepared to do so. To be successful, the parents, not the staff members on the health care team, must be ready.

Disclosers were also more cohesive than nondisclosers. Disclosers scored at least one standard deviation higher than the "normal family" mean for cohesion that was given in the scale's manual [Moos & Moos 1993]; the nondisclosers scored right in the vicinity of normal families (in contrast to distressed families). The reality of this disease, however, is that many of the children experience disruption and distress in their lives as they are shuttled between relatives and other care providers while their parents are ill, and basic needs such as food and shelter cannot always be met. In addition, secrecy may already be the norm in the family due to undisclosed paternity, previous history of drug use, previous undisclosed sexual relationships, and/or homosexuality. All of these factors could significantly affect the degree of cohesion that the family experiences. Regardless of how cohesive the family may be, helping the parent to establish open communication, pre- and post-disclosure of the diagnosis, is critical. Feelings of shame should be diminished while an atmosphere of trust and acceptance should be enhanced. The parent-child relationship will be strengthened only when the children feel they can trust their parents to be honest with them and in turn, the parents can recognize and empathize with their children's feelings of pain, sadness, and uncertainty.

Limitations, Clinical Implications, and Directions for Future Research

Clearly, one of the major limitations of this study was the small number of HIV-infected parents with biological children who participated; therefore, these results should be considered preliminary. The sample was so small because many of the children that come to our clinic are cared for by foster or adoptive parents or extended family members. This is not uncommon in the AIDS epidemic; it has been projected that by the year 2000, the number of motherless children and adolescents (due to maternal HIV) in the United States will exceed 80,000 [Levine 1993]. Future research would benefit from attempting to assess HIV-infected parents at an earlier point in time. In addition, Caucasian women were overrepresented in the study group. Differences in disclosure styles among parents of different races, ages, and cultural backgrounds, as well as between genders, should be considered in future studies when larger samples are available.

With acknowledgment of these limitations, the findings presented here have important clinical and research implications. The study confirmed that a great deal of secrecy and stigma still surround an AIDS diagnosis. Children who have been informed of their parents' HIV status, especially those children who are then asked to keep the diagnosis a secret, must be monitored to assess for changes in their psychological functioning. The present study indicated that these children were both concerned and sad after learning that their parents (and in this case, themselves) had HIV. It would be important to determine if a clinical picture of anxiety and/or depression develops, or whether the child's response is perhaps a short-term adaptive reaction to being given emotionally charged information. All of the respondents who had disclosed their diagnosis to their children reported being satisfied with their decision to do so, and they were also significantly less depressed than the nondisclosers. This could possibly indicate that disclosure is a process that contributes to psychological well-being. Conversely, there were clearly some negative implications described as well. These were evidenced by three parents reporting that their lives had worsened since the disclosure took place.

Indeed, the decision whether or not to disclose one's diagnosis to one's children is a powerful and personal decision. Parents must be afforded the time to make the decision. They also should be encouraged to explore both the positive and negative sequalae that might ensue. Health care providers should be sensitive to the individual needs of each family so that they can be supportive of the family before, during, and following the disclosure process (see figure 1).

Given the growing number of children who are faced with an HIV-infected parent and the relative lack of research in this area, many questions pertaining to disclosure remain to be answered. Each parent will disclose his or her diagnosis in a style that is comfortable for him or her. Examination of disclosure styles and the effect that different styles may have on both planning for the future and the child's ability to comprehend and cope with the diagnosis would be important. A number of questions can be asked in future research. Do parents who disclose their diagnosis to their children soon after the diagnosis is made make permanency plans earlier than parents who do not share the diagnosis with their chil-

FIGURE 1

Guiding a Family Through the Disclosure Process

As child welfare professionals, there are a number of factors to keep in mind when helping families throughout the disclosure process:

- Differences among diseases are not understood by the preschool child.
- The school-age child often asks a barrage of questions.
- The preadolescent and adolescent child will ask more sophisticated questions related to how the disease was acquired. One should be prepared to answer these questions before disclosing the diagnosis.
- Talking to children about a parent's HIV illness takes preparation.
- When parents talk about whether or not they want to share the diagnosis with their children, it is important to listen since this is a subject they do not often discuss with many people.
- Disclosure is a process that usually takes place over time—one can't expect children to understand all aspects of a parent's illness after one discussion.
- Parents may seek reassurance from the child welfare worker that they have made the right decision by disclosing or not disclosing the diagnosis to their child(ren). Although the worker may have a strong opinion regarding whether or not the child(ren) should be informed of the diagnosis, disclosure is a very personal decision. The professionals in the parent's life must not be judgmental.
- The impact of the diagnosis may take the child weeks to years to absorb. Remember to be where the child is at. If the child has specific questions, answer them. Let the child know that no matter how difficult the subject matter, he or she can always ask questions or share feelings. Be careful, however, not to provide more information than the child wants or is prepared for.
- Trust between the parent and child should always be the highest priority.

dren for some time or not at all? Is there a difference in the quality of life of the parents and/or the life expectancy of those parents who disclosed their diagnosis to their children as compared with those who did not? Is there an "ideal" age range when the children should be informed? Children in this study learned about their own diagnosis at the same time that they learned about their parents' diagnosis. Is there a difference in the reactions of HIV-infected children versus non-HIV-infected children to learning their parents' diagnosis? Do HIV-infected children feel a bond with their parents or feel less alone because they are living with the same disease? Do non-HIV-infected children feel left out because they do not have HIV or are they relieved to know that they are healthy? Parents who are living with HIV are increasingly diverse in terms of their age, family heritage, belief systems, economic circumstances, and geographic location [Draimin 1995]. How do all of these factors affect disclosure and the long-term emotional health of the children? Are the important variables associated with a positive psychological outcome related to the timing of the diagnosis disclosure, or perhaps more dependent on the quality of communication after the disclosure takes place?

Since disclosure is a lifelong process where one comes to terms with one's HIV status and its medical and social implications, research designs must allow for full exploration of a family's experiences, fears, and concerns [Lipson 1994]. Such information may not be able to be gathered sufficiently in a one-time, standardized interview. The use of both prospective and retrospective interviews, where parents are interviewed before and after disclosure, could provide essential information about the disclosure process. Longitudinal studies are important for assessing changes in psychological functioning over time and should include quantitative as well as in-depth qualitative methodology. Studies examining the effect that disclosure versus nondisclosure has on the parent-child bond, the mourning process, and the child's communication with others, would also be instrumental. Much can be learned from the individuals who face this disease and many of these individuals are eager to share their stories. It is important that their stories be heard. To do that, each study must be designed to take into consideration the complexities of this disease and the lives of those it affects. ◆

References

Barrera, M., & Ainley, S. (1983). The structure of social support: A conceptual and empirical analysis. *Journal of Community Psychology, 11*, 133–143.

Beck, A. T. (1967). *Depression, clinical, experimental and theoretical aspects*. New York: Harper.

Centers for Disease Control and Prevention. (1996a). *HIV/AIDS Surveillance Report, 8(2),* 12.

Centers for Disease Control and Prevention. (1996b). Personal communication. *CDC AIDS Hotline.*

Derlega, V. J., Lovejoy, D., & Winstead, B. A. (in press). Personal accounts of disclosing and concealing HIV-positive test results: Weighing the benefits and risks. In V. J. Derlega & A. Barbee (Eds.), *HIV infection and social interaction.* Newbury Park, CA: Sage Publications.

Draimin, B. (1995). A second family? Placement and custody decisions. In S. Geballe, J. Gruendel, & W. Andiman (Eds.), *Forgotten children of the AIDS epidemic* (pp. 125–139). New Haven, CT: Yale University Press.

Grollman, E. A. (1995). Grieving children: Can we answer their questions? In J. Doka (Ed.), *Children mourning, mourning children.* (pp. 17–27). Washington, DC: Hospice Foundation of America.

Harter, S. (1985). *Manual for the self-perception profile for children.* Denver, CO: University of Denver.

Harter, S. (1988). *Manual for the self-perception profile for adolescents.* Denver, CO: University of Denver.

Hays, R. B., McKusick, L., Pollack, L., Hilliard R., Hoff, C., & Coates, T. J. (1993). Disclosing HIV seropositivity to significant others. *AIDS, 7,* 425–431.

Husband, E., & Broaddhus, D. A. (1984). Children's books and stories as therapeutic metaphors: An intervention with seriously ill children. *Peodovita, 1,* 17–21.

Levine, C. (1993). *A death in the family: Orphans of the HIV epidemic.* New York: United Hospital Fund.

Lipson, M. (1994). Disclosure of diagnosis to children with Human Immunodeficiency Virus or Acquired Immunodeficiency Syndrome. *Journal of Developmental and Behavioral Pediatrics, 15,* S61–S65.

Moos, R. H., & Moos, B. S. (1993). *Family environment scale manual* (2nd ed.). Palo Alto, CA: Consulting Psychologists Press, Inc.

Ott, R. L. (1993). *An introduction to statistical methods and data analysis (4th ed.).* Belmont, CA: Duxbury Press.

Pennells, M., & Smith, S. C. (1995). *The forgotten mourners: Guidelines for working with bereaved children.* London: Jessica Kingsley Publishers, Ltd.

Pliskin, M., Farrell, K., Crandles, S., & DeHovitz, J. (1993). Factors influencing HIV positive mothers' disclosure to their non-infected children. *International Conference on AIDS, 9(2)*, 898.

Sigelman, C. K., & Shaffer, D. R. (1995). *Life-span human development* (2nd ed.). Pacific Grove, CA: Brooks/Cole Publishing Company.

Spinetta, J., & Deasy-Spinetta, P. (1981). *Living with childhood cancer.* St. Louis, MO: C.V. Mosby.

Stambrook, M., & Parker, K. (1987). The development of the concept of death in childhood: A review of the literature. *Merrill-Palmer Quarterly, 33*, 133–157.

Wiener, L. S., Battles, H. B., Heilman, N., Sigelman, C. K., & Pizzo, P. A. (1996). Factors associated with disclosure of diagnosis to children with HIV/AIDS. *Pediatric AIDS and HIV infection: Fetus to adolescent*, 7(5), 310–324.

Wiener, L. S., Heilman, N., & Battles, H. B. (in press). Psychosocial considerations of public disclosure of HIV for children. In V. Derlega & A. Barbee (Eds.), *Social interaction and HIV infection*. Newbury Park, CA: Sage.

Wilcoxon, F., & Wilcox, R. A. (1964). *Some rapid approximate statistical procedures*. Pearl River, NY: Lederle Laboratories.

3 Parental Loss Due to HIV: Caring for Children as a Community Issue—The Rochester, New York Experience

Susan Taylor-Brown, Judith Ann Teeter, Evelyn Blackburn, Linda Oinen, and Lennard Wedderburn

The number of children in the United States who will lose a parent to AIDS is increasing. Permanency planning to help families affected by AIDS includes case management, mental health, medical care, child welfare, and legal services. These services are provided by a number of different professions, and have largely been reactive and noncoordinated. This article presents the efforts of one community in a midsize city to develop and implement a multidisciplinary coordinated plan for providing services to children affected by the illness or death of a parent from HIV/ AIDS.

Susan Taylor-Brown, Ph.D., M.P.H., ACSW, is Chair, Health Care Concentration, Syracuse University School of Social Work, Syracuse, NY. Judith Ann Teeter, J.D., is Staff Attorney, Volunteer Legal Services Project, Rochester, NY. Evelyn Blackburn, CSW, is Director, Community Services, Community Health Network, Rochester, NY. Linda Oinen, CSW, is Administrative Caseworker, Monroe County Department of Social Services, Rochester, NY. Lennard Wedderburn, CSW, is Case Manager, Community Health Network, Rochester, NY.

As the AIDS epidemic continues, the impact of HIV/AIDS on infected parents and their children has become an expanding crisis with catastrophic consequences for families and the communities in which they live. Michaels and Levine [1992] estimate conservatively that as many as 125,000 children in the United States will lose their parents to HIV/AIDS by the year 2000. In New York State, HIV/AIDS now surpasses any other single cause of death for women 25 to 44 years of age [RATFA 1997]. Current estimates are that by the end of this decade, 58,000 children will have been orphaned in New York State by maternal death from HIV/AIDS [Working Committee on HIV, Children, and Families 1996].

New York State's Working Committee on HIV, Children and Families [1996] projects that 500 children will experience maternal loss from HIV/AIDS in the Rochester, New York region by the year 2000. Local estimates from experts in the social services and medical communities put the number of children closer to 1,000. The majority of these children are not infected with HIV [RATFA 1997].

As dramatic as the sheer numbers are, the destructive impact that HIV/AIDS is having on families, children, and communities of color is even more dramatic. By far, the majority of children who will lose a parent to AIDS—90%—will be African American and Latino [Committee on HIV, Children, and Families 1996]. In the African American and Latino communities, informal adoption by relatives (usually grandparents and aunts) is common; these relatives often care for children whose parents die or are unable to take care of them. In creating any kind of workable approach to caring for HIV-affected children, the informal placement systems and other support networks that exist in the African American and Latino communities must be recognized and supported. Additionally, any coordinated approach must develop culturally competent strategies for meeting the needs of children of all racial and ethnic backgrounds.

This article addresses the myriad challenges involved in mounting a community response to meet the permanency planning needs of affected children. Since the number of affected children in all areas is on the rise, it is essential that the impediments to the planning process be understood and solutions pursued with a comprehensive, multidisciplinary approach.

Rochester, located in western New York State, and a nonepicenter of the pandemic, typifies the challenges of "second wave" cities. Nonepicenter areas such as Rochester are eligible for fewer resources to assist in permanency planning, and face unique obstacles in comparison with service providers in the epicenters, such as New York City. AIDS is still heavily stigmatized in small cities, and there is a conspiracy of silence among family members and other caregivers about drug use and HIV/AIDS.

Developing comprehensive policy in a relatively small community, however, has certain advantages. Because the number of providers of social services, case management, medical care, and legal services in Rochester is limited, they have been able to come together to develop and then implement a five-year plan to respond to the needs of dependent children affected by HIV/AIDS. This committee of the Rochester Area Task Force on AIDS (RATFA) is a multidisciplinary group; its goal is to draw broad public support to the problem of providing services to affected children.

One of the group's strategies is to target services by using a public health approach, that is, by identifying the population of affected children as the recipients of needed communitywide services. This is in contrast to looking at the problem from the point of view of individual providers targeting services to individual clients or patients, or targeting the services to parents with HIV. By using a public health approach, we hope to provide a variety of services that stabilize families beginning at any point in the continuum, from the parent's diagnosis through the successful placement of the child in alternative care.

The Effect on Children of Parental Loss from HIV/AIDS

AIDS affects all family members. The possibility of premature death is an overwhelming challenge for any parent to contemplate, and this threatening loss is compounded by the stigma attached to HIV disease in our society. The impact of HIV disease on the lives of children is one of the epidemic's most tragic aspects. Although some children are themselves infected, most often a child's life is affected because of either one parent's or both parents' HIV infection; this is compounded when other family members are similarly infected.

These children experience multiple losses, with few resources to help them deal with bereavement and its repercussions. They face the threat and reality of family disruption, their parent's illness and eventual death, possible separation from their siblings, the necessity of adapting to new caregivers and new surroundings, and the loss of financial and emotional supports. New caregiver families often lack financial resources to care for children, and the children may be pushed into out-of-home care, and left financially destitute and emotionally troubled. Unfortunately, some youngsters, particularly adolescents, remain completely outside of the care system.

All of these losses are exacerbated by the complex interrelationships of HIV and poverty and drug use. Mistrust and fear of the legal system (or other government intervention) also hinder permanency planning efforts. In particular, parents whose histories include substance abuse and prostitution may fear that their children will be removed from their families.

The best environment for a child to deal with these crippling losses is an extended family situation, where the child is familiar with the caregiver and the caregiver is emotionally bound to the child. Caregiver relatives, however, may be unwilling to care for children from HIV-affected families. Also, extended family members may be in need of financial assistance to take on the care of additional family members; this assistance is often either unavailable or is substantially lower than that available in the traditional out-of-home care system.

The Permanency Planning Process

Dealing with the needs of surviving children under crisis conditions creates an urgent need to assist many parents infected with

HIV as they approach the later stages of illness, often without having begun to plan for the care of their children. Urgent help is also necessary to stabilize the new caregiver home that the child will enter, so as to avoid the need for out-of-home care.

Permanency planning is an ongoing process. It should include legal assistance with custody arrangements and the provision of a range of social support services. These services have to be provided to existing families, as well as to new families who will take over the care of the children when their parents are no longer able to do so. The necessary services include therapeutic counseling, support groups, and other mental health services for all family members; financial support to help new caregiver families through the transition period and to help all HIV-affected families maintain family stability; and advocacy for laws that provide quick and efficient ways of transferring legal custody or guardianship of children to new caregiver families when appropriate, but not before such transfers are needed.

Permanency planning has traditionally been viewed as a parent-centered activity. As it continues to evolve, people in the field are conceptualizing future planning as a child-centered, family-focused continuum. This has special relevance to HIV-infected parents because the majority do not make permanency plans for their children prior to their death. Thus, services to help with planning must begin at the time the parent is diagnosed, and continue beyond the time that the child is successfully placed, which frequently occurs after parental death. The services should follow the child until a guardianship arrangement is made; this is the safety net that we must give children. By and large, ongoing monitoring of guardianship arrangements resulting from AIDS-related parental death is currently nonexistent.

At the same time that the definition of permanency planning is being refocused and expanded, the approach to permanency planning is shifting from being considered a family-specific matter to a communitywide problem, requiring a community response. In Rochester, efforts are being targeted toward developing coordinated and collaborative arrangements among and between existing providers. These efforts are not limited to AIDS-specific service providers; they extend to existing human service and community leaders, such as religious leaders.

Providing Communitywide, Child-Centered Permanency Planning Services

In general, services related to permanency planning have sprung up in a fragmented and reactive manner. The idea of a coordinated approach is to provide the same spectrum of services to all HIV-infected parents or affected children, no matter the point at which they enter the service delivery system.

As noted previously, a public health approach to permanency planning views it as a population-based planning situation (which defines the service recipients as "all parents living with HIV who have dependent children") rather than reacting to the needs of individual cases. This broad-based approach, it is hoped, will mobilize the community to respond systemically rather than idiosyncratically. To develop a community approach, RATFA convened the subcommittee, Children and Families Affected by HIV/AIDS (CAFAA), to develop a plan for the regional five-year report and to work toward implementing the community interventions where outlined. The subcommittee represents the key medical, legal, social service, and community-based AIDS agencies, and the group has benefited from working together toward this common goal. This forum is useful for addressing the service providers' concerns and difficulties about working together to improve situations for affected families. It is easy to criticize the response of either another agency or the community to this need because of the reality that the responses to affected children are not adequate. It is harder but more rewarding to work collaboratively to enhance the overall community response.

The subcommittee's report is part of the five-year plan, and the subcommittee is collaborating on the delivery of the plan, which includes holding community forums to highlight the needs of HIV-affected families. Engagement of religious leaders is one of the top priorities and efforts are under way to involve them. Religious leaders were invited to a legislative breakfast and a general RATFA meeting on permanency planning, and further discussions of the service needs of families are planned.

The subcommittee has recognized several primary considerations as necessary for stabilizing children's lives:

1. Loss, rather than HIV, is the core concern in permanency planning.
2. Most parents, whether HIV infected or not, seldom make legal permanency plans for their children.
3. Fiscal constraints are obstacles to the appropriate delivery of services.
4. Permanency planning services must be expanded and reconceptualized, using the family as the focus, not just the HIV-infected parent.
5. Services must be provided in a culturally relevant manner. They must be extended beyond the initial placement of the children for a sufficient period of time following parental death to assure that the new family is stable.

Cultural Competence

As noted, 90% of the children affected by HIV/AIDS are from communities of color. Services must be accessible and acceptable to the African American and Latino communities. Services should also provide necessary spiritual, emotional, and financial support to surviving children. Specific historical relationships between communities of color and both medical and child welfare services must be considered in developing the contemporary response to affected children. Stigmatization of HIV disease in the African American community is widening, and many people continue to perceive HIV as a disease of gay Caucasian men. The African American and Latino communities have viewed the treatments for HIV disease with suspicion and distrust. The unfortunate legacy of the Tuskeegee study has permeated HIV care since its onset.*

* The study, which lasted over 40 years, involved African American men with syphilis. During the course of the study, they were told that their disease was being treated,

Currently, there is extraordinary confusion over the disparate views that people hold about HIV infection. For example, while many people still see HIV as a death sentence, others have been led to believe that protease inhibitors can cure HIV or keep it from progressing. This latter belief is exemplified by a recent quote by Magic Johnson's wife, who believes that he is cured: "He is still taking medication, but there is no virus in his blood" [Randolph 1997]. Such an optimistic view of HIV treatment may lead parents with HIV to think that planning is unnecessary.

The child welfare system has also had a problematic relationship in serving communities of color. Historically, African American children have not been well served by the child welfare system [Taylor-Brown et al. 1992]. The unresponsiveness of child welfare to the needs of African American children has caused many communities to use informal adoption as an alternative to out-of-home care within the system. Hill [1997] described informal adoption as an informal social service network that has been integral to the African American community since slavery. When relatives are unable or unwilling to raise orphaned children, however, there is an increase in out-of-home nonrelative care due to child welfare placements in family foster or adoptive homes.

The church, traditionally a source of strength in rallying the African American community to respond to adversity, has experienced limited success in relation to HIV. As a result, HIV continues to be highly stigmatized, and many parents who would normally turn to the church for comfort, support, and solace are reluctant to do so for fear of rejection. Many parents try to hide their diagnosis, or tell others that they have "cancer," which is perceived as more socially acceptable. The "One Church One Child" campaign to care for orphaned children has not been widely adopted. Ongoing efforts to

when treatment was actually being withheld [Jones 1981]. Not only were the men infected, many of their wives became infected as well. As a logical consequence of such deception, there is now is an ongoing tension and well-founded mistrust of Western medicine within the African American community. President Clinton, on behalf of the government, finally formally apologized to the survivors in May 1997.

involve religious leadership are essential for the success of permanency planning [Taylor-Brown et al. 1992].

Based on this historical reality, we must recognize the distrust that African Americans have of the medical, child welfare, and legal systems, and be sensitive to that distrust in offering culturally relevant permanency planning services. If we expect communities of color to access services, service providers must be able to explain the services in a context that makes sense to African Americans, Latinos, and all other cultural, racial, and ethnic groups. Too often, the cultural component is not fully understood, explored, or appreciated by the practitioners providing care. When people of color interact with Western health care systems, their cultural values related to health, illness, and help-seeking are often at variance with the values of the dominant system [Dalton 1991]. Wright et al. [1996] call for the validation of these feelings and the acknowledgment that biases do exist in our agencies.

These issues are central to the work of CAFAA. The committee comprises key service providers, with particular attention to the inclusion of advocates from the community. The original group is expanding to enhance the involvement of those affected. For example, it has come to light that mothers with infected children feel that there are not sufficient psychosocial supports for them or their children. As a result, they are becoming involved.

The committee meetings exemplify the challenges of working through mistrust. It is one thing to say "acknowledge the mistrust," but it is another to actually work through it. Experience suggests that providers frequently experience their own mistrust of other providers, in a parallel manner, as do family members dealing with the system. By meeting together and planning services, committee members are able to bring problems to the forefront and discuss them. What might appear to members of the community as agency unresponsiveness may, in fact, be regulatory restriction. The group is advocating to end these obstructions, enhance service delivery, and develop productive strategies.

Overview of Providers Addressing Permanency Planning with Affected Families

Second-wave cities are characterized by limited funding opportunities, which frequently result in the fragmentation of services. Agencies may develop overlapping services (e.g., case management) in some areas, while gaps remain in other services (e.g., parent support groups). The experiences of the central permanency planning providers are highlighted below to share the lessons learned thus far, with respect to (1) permanency planning legal services, (2) the role of medical social workers in permanency planning, and (3) the role of the child welfare system in permanency planning.

*Permanency Planning Legal Services**

In Rochester, the Volunteer Legal Services Project of Monroe County, Inc. (VLSP) receives funding from the New York State Department of Health AIDS Institute to provide permanency planning legal services to families affected by HIV/AIDS. Clients are eligible if a child has been in any way affected by a parent's illness or death from HIV/AIDS, and if the service will stabilize any aspect of the child's life. The grant pays for a half-time staff attorney. By comparison, many New York City programs include funding for social workers.

Legal Options for Custody Planning. In 1992, New York State passed a standby guardianship law, which enables a parent suffering from either a "progressively chronic illness" or an "irreversibly fatal illness" to plan the future care of her or his children without having to give up parental rights. This law was passed in response to the HIV epidemic and the possibility of a large number of children being orphaned with no plans made for their future. In most cases, standby guardianship is the best permanency planning option. All other permanency planning

* The author of this section, Judith Teeter, is a half-time staff attorney for VSLP.

options require parents to give up some or all of their parental rights while still alive, which has been an obstacle to planning for many parents. Other options include informal placement with friends or relatives, guardianship by petition or by will, custody proceedings, family foster care, or adoption.*

Legal Services Provided. Typically, once clients have understood the legal options available, they select standby guardianship. Common problems encountered within this legal vehicle include: how to give notice to absent fathers, and how to proceed if the father is unknown or if his whereabouts are unknown; procedural issues relating to appointing as guardian a Puerto Rico resident; legal questions of immigration status for either the proposed guardian or the client; procedural issues about whether co- or successor guardians can be appointed; and jurisdictional issues when the client and the guardian live in different states.

The major legal service requested by clients, other than custody planning, is help with obtaining Supplemental Security Income (SSI)—most commonly making appeals on denials of reconsideration. In addition, the service helps clients with obtaining public assistance; accessing other benefits such as Supplemental Security Disability Income (SSDI) survivors' benefits; housing; family law matters, including custody, visiting, divorce, child support, and establishing paternity; and permanency planning arrangements such as guardianship, family foster care, and adoption.

Program Model. VLSP is a pro bono program: the private attorneys donate their time to VLSP and do all of the legal work on behalf of the clients. The staff attorney's duties include community outreach

---

* *Note*: There are many excellent discussions of the legal options available for parents with HIV/AIDS, including: Geballe, S., Toward a Child-Responsive Legal System, in S. Geballe, J. Gruendel, and W. Andiman (Eds)., (1995). *Forgotten Children of the AIDS Epidemic*, New Haven: Yale University Press; Pinott, M. (1994). *Custody and Placement: The Legal Issues*, and Herb, A. (1994). *The New York State Standby Guardianship Law: A New Option for Terminally Ill Parents*, in C. Levine and G. Stein (Eds)., *Orphans of the HIV Epidemic: Unmet Needs in Six Cities*, New York: United Hospital Fund; Cooper, E. (1992). *HIV-Infected Parents and the Law: Issues of Custody, Visitation and Guardianship*, in N. Hunter and W. Rubenstein (Eds)., *AIDS Agenda: Emerging Issues in Civil Rights*, New York: The New Press.

and education; client recruitment, screening, and intake; case follow-up and monitoring; volunteer lawyer recruitment, training, and mentoring; and program design and evaluation. The actual legal proceedings and ongoing legal counsel and advice are carried out or provided by volunteer attorneys matched with each client. Thus, although funding is provided only for a half-time staff attorney, the service can represent clients in up to 100 cases at any given time. The benefit for the cost is enormous.

This model also has a negative side, however. It requires additional work on the part of the client because she or he must be screened at VLSP, then make an appointment for an initial meeting with the volunteer lawyer. Such follow-through can prove to be overly demanding for a client who already feels overwhelmed by the process of making a plan for future custody. In tracking outcomes, we have found that the clients who do best in completing custody plans tend to be those who have had extensive involvement with either a social worker, case manager, or medical provider, and have had prior opportunities to thoroughly discuss the various aspects of permanency planning.

Client recruitment and retention would likely be improved by having a social services component within the project. Clients often need the buffer of a social service provider or case manager to approach the complexities of permanency planning. Due to the difficulty of dealing with the psychosocial intensities in these cases, clients are more comfortable when they have experienced some prior therapeutic work before beginning to grapple with the legal process.

Since this type of work is so heavily oriented toward social services, the work of volunteer attorneys must be carefully integrated with the work of social workers and case managers within the community. The staff attorney is used to coordinate all services to clients. While this has improved services to clients, and helped volunteer attorneys understand some of the more prevalent psychosocial elements involved in working with HIV-affected families, the success rate varies with the rate of involvement of the client's particular social worker or case manager. The presence of a social worker on staff at the program would contribute to the achievement of more consistent results with the same work.

Trends in Readiness of Clients to Initiate Planning. The readiness of clients is extremely variable, and has had an important impact on the nature of our work. The no-show and no follow-through rate has been about 25% to 35%. Certain factors that have been identified help explain why clients might or might not complete a legal custody plan:

- The length of time clients have worked with a social worker to approach permanency planning favorably affects how well they will do in completing the legal process;
- The more ill the clients, the more likely they have been found to complete the process quickly (as a trend, healthier clients focus their energies on the other exigencies of everyday life—food, transportation, medical care, child care, housing—rather than on custody plans);
- The "cleaner" the family situation is (i.e., the clients are clear about their choice for guardian, the guardian is already involved with the children in some way, absent parents either consent or cannot be found, the extended family is supportive of the client and their children, etc.), the more likely the clients will finish the legal custody plan;
- The more recently a client has been involved with drugs, the less likely the client is to complete a custody plan, or even follow through with an initial meeting with the attorney.

Trends in Outcomes of Planning/Types of Plans/New Caregivers. Although standby guardianship is the most common of the legal procedures used for permanency planning, recent trends in choosing other procedures have been noted:

- In a number of cases, the client's children are already living with the proposed guardian (usually the mother or sister of the client); in these cases it is more typical that the client will choose a straight guardianship.

- In a few cases, clients are already working within the out-of-home care system with potential adoptive families. Advocacy for these clients ensures that they understand what is happening in the process, and that their needs are met in terms of continuing visiting and contact with their children.
- In a number of cases, the client has died while the process of pursuing a standby guardian has been under way; in most of these cases the proposed guardian continues the work of obtaining letters of guardianship.
- The vast majority of new caregivers for clients thus far have been the clients' mothers. Next is a sister, and third is a partner, who has typically been the father of the youngest child but not of the older children.
- Many family relationships are complicated by loss and grief, poverty, drug use, felony history, special needs of children, and family instability. Often, the client simply does not have the emotional resources to consider the future at all.
- Race, ethnicity, and culture all have major roles in the different types of decisions different parents will make regarding the care of their children.

Lessons Learned. Lawyers are typically not prepared to provide all the advice clients need on making future custody plans for children. Such work involves a knowledge of subjects that come under the disciplines of law, medicine, and social work. As Draimin [1995] states: "Ideally, each parent who begins to explore custody options for her children would have the help of a multidisciplinary team, including at least a mental health professional, an attorney, and an entitlement specialist, all of whom are trained in family therapy, child development, custody law, and the HIV disease process." Quite clearly, the reality of this type of work does not yet approach that ideal.

Our experience has taught us that, when at all possible, legal services programs should be provided with funding for a social services component within the project. This will enable the legal services project to do additional ongoing direct work with clients, and to ensure that clients follow through with the legal work and complete custody plans.

The Role of Medical Social Workers in Permanency Planning*

A major impediment to service development for HIV-affected children is the impression that few children are being affected. Significantly, most HIV medical centers are not monitoring the status of dependent children unless they are HIV infected. It would be a major step forward if a systemwide approach to developing data on HIV-affected children were implemented at all medical and social service centers.

Even when affected children are considered in data collection, too often questions are directed only to mothers in HIV care, not fathers—a serious problem. Of course, fathers being treated for HIV/AIDS also have dependent children, and, even when fathers are not custodial parents, the loss of either parent is devastating to children and affects their emotional and financial well-being.

Service providers in the medical setting often focus on the complexities of HIV medical care to the exclusion of psychosocial considerations. Within the context of providing medical services, recognition of the importance of planning for the future can help focus community services for affected children. Since medical care is almost always a parent's first entry into the vast system of HIV-related services, the best opportunity to broach the subject of permanency planning may be with the HIV care team. Medical providers, however, tend to see the individual's psychosocial needs only as they relate to medical compliance. This leaves the entire subject of planning to the uncertain possibility that clients may become involved with social workers or case managers who can help them through this intensely emotional ordeal.

Social workers in HIV medical care centers have a unique opportunity to reach out to parents to help them plan for their children's future. This outreach effort represents an addition to

* The author of this section, Evelyn Blackburn, is the Director of Community Services at Community Health Network in Rochester, New York.

traditional case management and appears to hold promise for affected children and their parents.

Program Model. The Community Health Network (CHN) is a freestanding, nonprofit medical outpatient clinic in Rochester, New York, dedicated to treating persons who are HIV positive. CHN opened in 1989 under a medical director. The clinic initially began serving the male gay population. It was not long, however, before women and minorities became part of the patient population. The Community Services staff, consisting of five social workers/case managers, completes an initial psychosocial assessment for each patient.

The needs of affected children are becoming increasingly prominent in these assessments. During the past two years it has become clear that, while the number of infected or affected children of the female patients were being tracked, no male patient, regardless of sexual orientation, had been asked if he was the custodial or noncustodial parent of infected or affected children. A retrospective chart review of active male patients revealed that over 250 children were affected by their HIV/AIDS status, in addition to the 170 children of the female patients, for a current total of 420 children affected by HIV/AIDS at this one treatment facility.

Male patients often fear that if they disclose that they are noncustodial parents, CHN will report them to the Department of Social Services for child support payments. Once the social worker reassures patients that the information will not be released to an outside agency, they are willing to provide the information about their children.

Social workers in medical settings can help parents explore planning for the future and link the parents to services. In a sense, parents are a captive audience. Although they are at CHN primarily to obtain medical care, it is easy for them to begin dealing there with planning since they do not have to travel to another agency to do so. Early referral efforts outside the agency were mainly unsuccessful. Many parents equated going to legal services with giving up on parenting, and with impending death. Efforts to "detoxify" the losses surrounding planning have increased parental willingness to explore the process of permanency planning. These efforts are presented as a way that parents can help shape their children's future. Psychoeducational group approaches appear to allow parents to accept their losses, and at the same time create an opportunity for peer support.

The clinic now offers a six-week psychoeducational support group called Capturing Memories. The group is open to anyone in the community who is HIV positive. Capturing Memories was developed to help parents support each other, and to preserve family memories for their children. The parents who participate are from various ethnic, cultural, and socioeconomic backgrounds. Including the concept of preserving family memories for children as part of the future care planning process lessens the pressure of the legal process on the parents and their fear of it. The group process also assists parents in becoming focused by helping them complete several different tasks that evolve naturally over the course of the group sessions.

In the first group session, parents receive a large notebook, which they can develop for each one of their children. The facilitator then reviews the purpose of the group, as well as the activities for each of the six weeks. Each parent then reads poems to set the mood of empowerment and allow the parents' voices to be heard [Gilligan 1982]. The video, *A Gift for My Children* [Castle Lane Production 1995] is then presented and discussed.

The facilitator then explains the concept of a genogram [McGoldrick & Gerson 1985], and the initial steps are taken to develop a three-generational genogram for each parent. During the next four weeks, the group members are encouraged to explore their family histories by talking with older family members, beginning journal writing or oral taping of family memories, and gathering family photos to build a photo album for each child. Group members are encouraged to share the information they have learned, as well as their family photos. The work on the genograms continues with the assistance of graduate social work students and/or peer educators who have completed the Capturing Memories group. Group members are also encouraged to bring in poems or stories that were important to them or are important to their children. The meaning of the poems and stories are explored and incorporated into their notebooks as part of the legacy the parents are preparing for their children.

The fifth session is devoted to videotaping for the purpose of leaving a remembrance videotape for each child. The camera is set up before the arrival of the parents. The facilitator presents an introduction to videotaping, and the camera runs continuously to help the parents feel comfortable before the camera. The group then discusses how to prepare to videotape [Taylor-Brown 1994] and the facilitator answers the parents' questions and makes each participant comfortable with the videotaping process.

During the sixth and final session, the VLSP attorney meets with the group in a relaxed, nonthreatening environment. This allows parents to have an initial exposure to the legal process of permanency planning in a neutral setting with other group members present for support. Many parents have similar questions for the lawyer, and they feel a sense of safety in posing their questions in the group setting. Clients then make individual appointments with the attorney if they wish.

Every parent is provided with a "legacy box" for each child to store the notebook, photos, videotape, genogram, and any additional memorabilia the parent may wish to add. Evaluations are also completed and appointments are scheduled for individual recording sessions of remembrance videotapes. Parents are welcome to come back if they have new information to add to their genogram or need assistance to complete their legacy project.

Lessons Learned. Each Capturing Memories group has developed its own characteristic strengths and weaknesses. The pilot group was all female. In the process of recapturing childhood experiences for their children, one parent remembered that as a ten-year old, she had been held at gunpoint and raped. Another parent remembered the severe physical abuse she and her siblings suffered from an alcoholic parent. Yet another parent learned that the man she thought had been her father for the past 34 years was not her father, and that she had several more brothers and sisters in another state. Imber-Black [1993] writes, "secrets enervate the rules of shame—rules that perpetuate the shame and bind family members in confusion, chaos, and growth-inhibiting relationships." Although painful for the participants, these events empowered the parents to take control of their lives, find their own voice, and move from being reactive victims to being able to repair some broken relationships or view their families from a different perspective.

Each group has also contained parents with limited educational backgrounds, learning disabilities, or neurological impairment from HIV. One parent told of how much he hated school, especially reading, and of how he struggled to write a full sentence. Yet he was able to speak eloquently to his beloved daughter on the tape recorder, and also on the videotape. His message to his daughter was clear and straightforward...how much he loved her, how sorry he felt for some choices that he made in his life, and how his recovery from drug addiction had given him specific goals for the remainder of his life, one day at a time, however long his life might be. Another parent, college educated, said, "I guess this had to hit me over the head...preparing my son's legacy. Now, when I can't sleep at night, I write and write and write to my son."

*The Role of the Child Welfare System in Permanency Planning**

The Monroe County Department of Social Services (MCDSS) in Rochester, a public agency, provides mandated services in the areas of child protection, out-of-home care, day care, and adult protection to the families of Monroe County. Its mission is to "help individuals and families to maximize self-reliance and independence during periods of financial, medical, or emotional need, thereby enhancing the quality of life of the whole community." The Service Division staff believes the whole community must accept responsibility for the welfare of its members, thus maintaining a focus on community collaboration.

---

* The author of this section, Linda Oinen, is an administrative caseworker in the Service Division of MCDSS.

Program Model. This public agency, like many others, was slow in its response to the HIV/AIDS epidemic. With growing awareness of the situation, MCDSS formed its own internal committee in 1989, in collaboration with the Monroe County Department of Health, to deal with HIV/AIDS concerns for its clients. This group met for two years in an effort to develop an HIV/AIDS policy. As the group worked to develop the policy, the staff's awareness also grew. In 1992, a Services supervisor was designated as a liaison to the Rochester Area Task Force on AIDS (RATFA). This was the beginning of MCDSS's formal involvement in community planning concerning the HIV/AIDS epidemic.

In September 1994, the author, a graduate social work student at Syracuse University, worked as a MCDSS foster care supervisor and was assigned to an internship at Community Health Network (CHN) in Rochester. The internship had two purposes: to enhance the relationship between the MCDSS and HIV/AIDS caregivers to better meet the needs of those affected or infected, particularly in relation to permanency planning, and to allow the social work student intern the opportunity to gain sufficient information about HIV/AIDS to be able to write an agency policy for MCDSS.

This cross-systems relationship gave MCDSS the ability to identify and overcome obstacles to service provision for its clients. As cases were identified where services were impeded, either in the DSS or the HIV/AIDS system of care, joint determinations were made of the best course of action for the clients. The VLSP lawyer working on permanency planning was also available to consult on these cases. Connections and relationships between MCDSS, the medical community, and the legal community enhanced the services available to clients. This cross-systems relationship also increased MCDSS's awareness of the specific needs of the HIV/AIDS populations. In 1996, an HIV/AIDS policy was developed for MCDSS.

Lessons Learned. HIV-infected clients generally do not approach MCDSS to make permanency plans for their children, unless they have no family members available to become guardians. This population presents complex and unique needs. For example, although mothers often do not wish their children to be placed with the father, MCDSS has to explore fathers as a potential placement resource unless there is a court order restricting such placement or a substantial reason not to. Moreover, identifying an appropriate placement is complicated. A family that would be interested in adopting in the future is ideal. The foster family would have to be a family who could make a long-term commitment to the children, but would also be available on an as-needed basis for shorter placements when the parent required hospitalization. Placing a child in family foster care in New York State is a legally cumbersome and often frightening process for people who are already coping with all of the emotional and medical ramifications of their illness. MCDSS's cross-systems approach helps to minimize blockages and to create successful plans for its families. In addition, MCDSS's presence in community collaborative relationships helps to dispel some of the myths about the DSS system, and encourages the formation of trusting relationships among providers.

The MCDSS staff also recognized the need to make supports available to families who are looking for informal placements with friends or relatives. MCDSS had developed a "relative resource guide" to give families the necessary information regarding what supports are available to them. Whenever possible, MCDSS works to keep children out of the foster care system. The amount that Monroe County pays to foster parents to care for a child is, however, significantly more than the amount the federal Temporary Assistance Program will pay for a relative to care for a child. This forces some children into the "system" who do not need to be there.

Asking parents to formalize permanency planning for their children while the parents are relatively healthy and of sound mind contradicts how most cultures value children. In America, the local county department of social services assigns a preventive worker when a child is reported at risk of abuse or neglect. Generally, if the case is founded for abuse or neglect, and a child's health or safety is at risk, the next step is the removal of the child to out-of-home care services. Now, as an option for permanency planning, if parents cannot locate a legal guardian for their child or children, they are being asked to voluntarily allow the out-of-home care system to assist them in preparing for their children to be adopted. This is a major shift for parents: previously dependent and fearful of the public social services system, they must now view the services that MCDSS can provide to them in a positive light.

There is still a long way to go to become fully responsive to the particular needs of HIV/AIDS-infected/affected individuals and the many other populations we are mandated to serve. Flexible placement resources that are available and willing to commit to meeting the needs of the HIV/AIDS population still need to be developed. Better linkages are needed with the federal public assistance programs so that adequate financial resources can be available to people outside of the foster care system. Finally, the multidisciplinary approach must be broadened so that all of the appropriate systems are working together, to maximize the limited resources available to best meet the complex needs of our families.

Conclusion

By applying a public health perspective to permanency planning, and by broadening the focus to planning for the future of the children, the community is responding more sensitively to the needs of HIV-affected children. Expanding the focus from a parent-centered activity to a family-centered activity where providers are committed to working with either parents or their children, at any point in the process from diagnosis to after parental death, we hope, will allow us to provide for more children. It is not acceptable to "lose" children to follow-up subsequent to parental death. Each community must develop an inclusive response to these members of the community. ◆

References

Castle Lane Productions. *A gift for my children: Families talk about custody planning*. Available from The Family Center, 66 Reade Street, New York, NY 10007.

Dalton, H. (1991). AIDS in blackface. In N. McKenzie (Ed.), *The AIDS reader: Social, political & ethical issues* (pp. 125–143). New York: Meridian.

Draimin, B. (1995). A second family? Placement and custody decisions. In S. Geballe, J. Gruendel, and W. Andiman (Eds.), *Forgotten children of the AIDS epidemic* (pp. 125–139). New Haven, CT: Yale University Press.

Families in Crisis. (1996). Report of the Working Committee on HIV, Children, and Families, a task force convened by the Federation of Protestant Welfare Agencies. Copies of the report may be obtained by calling 212/777–4800.

Gilligan, C. (1982). *In a different voice: Psychological theory and women's development*. Cambridge, MA: Harvard University Press.

Hill, R. (1977). *Informal adoption among black families*. Washington, DC: Urban League.

Imber-Black, E. (1993). *Secrets in families and family therapy*. New York: W.W. Norton & Company.

McGoldrick, M., & Gerson, R. (1985). *Genograms in family assessment*. New York: W.W. Norton & Company.

Michaels, D., & Levine, C. (1992). Estimates of the number of motherless youth orphaned by AIDS in the United States. *Journal of the American Medical Association, 268*, 3456–3461.

National Institute of Allergy and Infectious Disease. (1995, February). *Women and HIV infection*. Bethesda, MD: U.S. Public Health Service.

Randolph, L. (1997, April). Cookie Johnson or the Magic miracle: The lord has healed Earvin. *Ebony*, 72–76.

Rochester Area Task Force on AIDS (RATFA). (1997). *Five year plan for HIV/AIDS services*. Available from: Health Systems Agency, 1150 University Avenue, Rochester, NY 14607.

Taylor-Brown, S., & Wiener, L. (1994). Making videotapes of HIV-infected women for their children. *Families in Society*, 468–80.

Taylor-Brown, S., Wilczynski, C., Moore, E., & Cohen, F. (1992). Perinatal AIDS: Permanency planning for the African-American community. In J. Morales & M. Bok (Eds.), *Multicultural human services for AIDS treatment and prevention: Policy, perspective, and Planning* (pp. 85–105). Binghamton, NY: Haworth Press, Inc.

Wright, E., Blackburn, E., & Taylor-Brown, S. (1996, Fall). African American women still remain invisible: Are social workers doing enough? Clinical Cultural Competence Issues. *NSWAN Readings & Writings, 1*(3), 49–62.

4 Custody Planning with HIV-Affected Families: Considerations for Child Welfare Workers

Sally Mason

Most of the literature on permanency planning is based on the assumption that HIV-infected parents have custody of their children. A growing number of children entering child protective services, however, have an HIV-infected parent. Whether reunification or adoption is the permanency goal, these parents are concerned about their children's future after the parents' death. This article is drawn from research on custody planning with HIV-infected parents, from clinical literature and experience, and from a training curriculum for child welfare workers developed and implemented by the author. The lessons learned about custody planning with HIV-involved families are applied to practice with families who are involved with the state because of abuse or neglect of their children.

Sally Mason, Ph.D., is Assistant Professor for Clinical Social Work, Institute for Juvenile Research, Department of Psychiatry, University of Illinois at Chicago, Chicago, IL. *This manuscript is based in part on a training curriculum supported by Elizabeth Monk and the Illinois Department of Children and Family Services.*

Women represent one of the fastest growing groups of people infected with HIV [Hackl et al. 1997; Ickovics & Rodin 1992]. This shift in the demographics of the HIV epidemic presents a new set of challenges to the child welfare system. Earlier in the epidemic, child welfare professionals had to move quickly to meet the needs of infected children. In more recent years, public health officials and women's rights advocates have refocused the issue on women with HIV and their children—children who are not infected but are *affected* by their parent's illness. Professionals have responded with innovative programs and research into the custody planning needs of HIV-infected parents [Levine 1995]. The literature and many of the programs, however, focus chiefly on women who have custody of their children and are not involved with child protective services.

The needs of HIV-affected families are similar to those of other families in the child welfare system. HIV-affected families, however, have some special needs related to stigmatization and the disease process. Whether reunification or surrender is the permanency goal for these families, child welfare workers have , at least, the opportunity to introduce the idea of long-term planning to HIV-infected parents and, at best, to help parents put a plan in place in case they die before their children are grown.

Background

In 1996, at least one out of every four persons who tested HIV positive was female [Centers for Disease Control 1996]; some experts say the rate may be as high as one in three. Women of color make up the majority of women who are infected—in 1996, 57% of women diagnosed with AIDS were African American, and 19% were Hispanic [Centers for Disease Control 1996]. Though the public still believes injected drug use is the main route of transmission for women, in 1996, heterosexual transmission accounted for a slightly higher percentage of cases in women than injected drug use [Centers for Disease Control 1996].

As the number of HIV-infected women increases, so does the number of HIV-affected children. Michaels and Levine [1992] estimate that 80,000 children and adolescents in the U.S. will lose a mother to AIDS by the year 2000. The increase in the number of infected women and affected children in the U.S. is reflected in the child welfare system. In the Illinois Department of Children and Family Services, the number of HIV-infected women has increased almost 250% since 1994 and more than 800% since 1991 [Monk 1997]. Many other cases are likely unreported; HIV-infected women are often reluctant to tell anyone, especially a child welfare worker.

Most of the children of these women are healthy; they do not have HIV. When one family member has HIV, however, everyone in the family is affected by the illness [Wilson 1995]. Children or extended family may exhibit similar feelings to the person with HIV, including guilt, anger, and fear [Bonuck 1993]. Children or relatives often live and mourn in secret, isolated from social support and formal services because of the stigma of HIV [Dane 1993; LSC and Associates 1994; Tiblier et al. 1989]. HIV-affected families are best served by programs that acknowledge the impact of HIV on every member of the family [Gruendel & Anderson 1995; Tiblier et al. 1989; Wilson 1995].

The traditional permanency planning literature is surprisingly lacking in content concerning the planning needs of parents with children who are affected by a terminal illness. One group that does have some characteristics in common with HIV-infected mothers are elderly parents of adult children with disabilities, especially developmental disabilities. Elderly parents are in a position to plan for dependent children because of the parent's impending death or physical deterioration. Investigations of the propensity of parents to plan indicate that most deal with the decision by not deciding [Heller & Factor 1988; Smith & Tobin 1989]. Substitute care is difficult to discuss, especially as the options are perceived as ugly and painful. The topic is avoided. Parents make no concrete plans or assume that children will live with a sibling or other relative [Heller & Factor 1988; Smith & Tobin 1989].

Studies of parents with HIV replicate this finding—HIV-infected mothers tend to not make plans [Gamble 1993]. Sometimes planning is thwarted because the mother has no potential caregiver in mind. In recent studies of HIV-positive mothers and their children, roughly a third of the women said they could not identify a future caregiver for their children [LSC and Associates 1994; Mason 1995]. Adolescents in these families may be even less likely to have plans in place than younger children [Draimin et al. 1992].

Sometimes, parents do not plan because planning is a painful reminder of death. Mothers with AIDS, however, have identified several advantages to planning: it relieves pressure on them as a parent, ensures a normal life for their children (including a smooth transition to a new home), and gives them and their children a choice in where the children will live; children will know that their mother cared enough to plan for them and will know where they are going [Mason 1995]. Planning has a potential positive psychological impact on the parents and their children.

Psychosocial Issues of HIV-Infected Parents and Children

Like other parents, mothers with HIV place great importance on their role as a parent [Florence et al. 1994; Hackl et al. 1997]. Mothers say that one of the first questions that pop into their heads when they find out they have HIV is "What will happen to my children?" [Mason 1995]. Finding someone to care for their children can be an intimidating process. Mothers would like someone who can take all of their children, if possible, and meet the special needs of each child [Draimin 1995; Mason 1995]. Most parents will only trust someone whom they have watched with their children over a long period of time. A mother's realization that she has no one in her circle of family or friends that she trusts is difficult to face [Draimin 1995]. Mothers with AIDS also fear that, even if they identify a potential caregiver, that person may change her or his mind about caring for the children after the mother's death [Mason 1995].

Mothers who plan to tell the children and potential caregivers about their HIV status may anticipate rejection or blame. They may fear that they cannot answer all of the children's questions and will also have to talk about how they contracted the disease [Tasker

1992]. Mothers want to protect their children; they fear that their children will not be able to keep the HIV secret and feel guilty about burdening them with such a secret.

A positive HIV test or an AIDS diagnosis is an abrupt reminder of mortality. Having to plan for the imminent future of one's children because of impending death means not seeing the children grown and not playing with grandchildren; it means knowing that the children may eventually call someone else "mother." A sense of urgency may inform a parent's relationships with children and extended family because of this realization of a shortened lifespan. The importance of the parent role becomes acute when a parent has HIV because time is of the essence. When asked about talking to her children, Nickie said:

> Oh, it's hard now, just every little subject, any little thing that comes up that you might want to teach your child or talk to your child about, wondering if you're gonna be there, you know, if you're not. Should I hurry up and write this down or do this? Constantly should I talk to them about this now or...? Where do you start and where do you relax? [Mason 1995]

Most importantly for the child welfare worker, parents of children in care may bring a sense of urgency to the child welfare bureaucracy. If reunification is the goal, the mother may want it to happen very quickly so she has more time with her children. If adoption is the goal, the mother may want the legal arrangements in place before she becomes severely ill or dies.

With the prospect of early death, the role of parent and the importance of children are amplified. The end of life is about taking stock—about reviewing what one has accomplished. For many parents, seeing their children healthy and happy provides proof that the parents were successful. Their children are seen as their legacy to the world. As the end of life is brought closer by a diagnosis, being a good parent takes on new importance.

Children have some important questions when they find out that a parent has HIV. The questions vary depending on the age and cognitive development of the child. Some themes are common, however: When will my parent die? What's going to happen to me? What is happening to my mother? Who can I tell about this? What should I tell them? Did I cause this? Will the same thing happen to me? What can I do to help? [Evans et al. 1994; McKelvy 1993]. Children experience worry, fear, anger, sadness, and confusion [McKelvy 1993]. They often cannot discuss their feelings directly but show their feelings through problems at school or at home, such as fighting, withdrawing, or difficulty in sleeping [Zayas & Romano 1994]. When the parent's illness or the future is not talked about, young children, especially, may make up their own answers to these questions—answers that contribute to their fear and misunderstanding [McKelvy 1993].

Planning

In in-depth interviews, mothers with AIDS identified a list of activities as key in the custody planning process [Mason 1995]. These activities apply to parents who are working toward reunification and to parents who are considering surrendering their rights so that someone else can adopt. The activities provide a framework for understanding the HIV-affected family's planning needs within the child welfare system and the child welfare worker's role in that process. Brief vignettes exemplify how some parents have handled the activities and how child welfare workers have played a part.

Identifying Permanent Caregivers

Parents begin this activity by thinking through their support networks to see whom they might trust with their children. They may have some particular characteristics in mind for a caregiver, such as religious beliefs, the number of other children in the home, or their children's preferences. After mentally screening the possibilities and choosing someone, the parents must then ask the potential caregiver to care for the children.

In a child protective case, the foster parent may be an option as a potential caregiver. HIV-infected parents may not have considered the foster parent in that role, especially if reunification has been the goal. Given the opportunity to meet and talk with a foster parent, however, an HIV-infected parent may choose the foster parent as the potential caregiver. Foster parents may be especially attractive as permanent caregivers if biological parents have observed them with their children and sense that they can trust the foster parents. To talk to the foster parent about permanently caring for her children, the biological mother needs access to that person. The caseworker is often the key to that access. The worker will have to assist with contact and may even facilitate the discussion.

> Karen, an HIV-infected mother, was about to be reunited with her children but was still concerned about a custody plan in the event of her death. She had no friends or relatives that she thought were appropriate caregivers. She spoke with the foster mother, who agreed to be the permanent caregiver if Karen died before the children were grown. Karen and the foster mother talk frequently on the phone and occasionally the foster mother, mother, and the children go on outings. The foster mother became, in essence, Karen's extended family.

If the mother does not want the foster parent as the potential caregiver and has no other options, then the worker's role may be to help the mother rebuild relationships with extended family members or identify other resources for adoption. Resources may be formal, such as adoption programs, or informal, such as churches and community groups.

Talking to Children about HIV Disease and Death

This activity entails the mother not only telling her children that she has HIV/AIDS and what that means, but also answering questions and trying to help the children sort through their feelings. Some mothers want help telling their children that they have HIV. Others have told their children but are looking for help with continuing discussions. Workers can model ways to discuss the subject and make sure parents are educated about each child's developmental stage. Parents have to know what a child can understand and what to expect in a reaction.

Parents may benefit from hearing that "disclosure" does not have to be an all or nothing process. Parents do not have to tell their children about their HIV status as soon as they know but can give them information at different points over time. A parent may first talk to her children when a significant event occurs, such as an opportunistic infection or receipt of an AIDS diagnosis. Asking the child's preferences for future caregivers is another opportunity to talk about HIV. A variety of opportunities will arise to have discussions with children, and each discussion can build on the last, providing increasingly specific information and answering additional questions the children may have. Draimin [1995] suggests avoiding the word "disclosure," which has a negative connotation. Instead, a worker should explore how the family talks about significant events in their lives and adapt a discussion of HIV to that context.

> Andrea was concerned because her children did not talk to her about her illness. She had told them that she had HIV but considered their initial reaction too tame. She felt they were holding their feelings inside. She was not sure that she knew enough about their developmental capacity to be of help to them. A multiple family support group of HIV-infected parents and their children provided education generally about children's reactions and developmental needs. The children had the opportunity to meet other children in similar situations. The group provided an ongoing forum for discussion as her health or the children's needs changed.

Some parents do not want their children to know that they have HIV. They may tell them they are ill but not name the disease or they may not tell them anything. Workers must respect the parents' decision and talk to the children about HIV only with the parents' permission. The worker can advise the parents, however, that children often know that something is wrong even if no one has told them—they see a parent taking pills, they go to the clinic with the parent, or they overhear whispered conversations [Tasker 1992]. If the subject is not discussed, children often make things up ("it's my fault") to help themselves deal with the uncertainty. For a parent to deny an illness sets up an atmosphere of mistrust and potential betrayal if the child finds out the truth.

> In a counseling session with Kerry and his father, Kerry was given the opportunity to ask his father anything he wanted to know about his father's HIV illness. Kerry's first question was, "Why didn't you trust me with the truth a long time ago?"

Workers can problem-solve with parents, educate parents about children's developmental capacity, educate children about HIV/AIDS, and refer the family to resources, such as family counseling or support groups. Workers can also become a member of a "safe" network of people that parents and children establish. The reality is that children face discrimination and rejection when they tell friends or schoolmates that their parent has HIV. If the children are to keep the secret, parents should identify a few key "safe" persons with whom the children can talk about their parent's illness.

Talking to Potential Caregivers about HIV

The parent's concern about telling the potential caregiver is similar to telling the children. Parents may face rejection or blame or they may have to answer questions about past behaviors that are stigmatizing, such as questions of drug use or sexual behavior. In many cases, the potential caregiver is a relative who is currently providing care for the children. Relatives are increasingly taking on the care of HIV-affected children, whether through formal or informal arrangements [Blanche et al. 1996; Draimin 1995]. Telling relative caregivers about his or her HIV status may jeopardize the parent's present relationship with the family as well as future plans for the children. Telling a relative/potential caregiver may also open the children to criticism or rejection. Relationships in the family may already be fraught with anger because of the parent's drug use or other strains on the family system [Burton 1992; Cates et al. 1990; Gruendel & Anderson 1995; Minkler et al. 1993]. The potential caregiver may at this point change her mind about caring for the children in the future. The parent must then start the process over and identify a new potential caregiver.

> Flora had not told her children or the kinship care providers that she had HIV. She was a recovering addict and active in the community doing prevention and peer education. She had recently made a TV public service message that would soon be aired. She admitted forcing herself into a position where she was going to have to tell her family, but did not know how to begin. Her relationship with the relative caregiver of her youngest children was difficult. The paternal grandmother "bad-mouthed" her in front of her children because of her past drug use. She was dreading telling the grandmother about her HIV status because of the impact it might have on her relationship with her children.

A child welfare worker could have helped her prepare to tell her family, facilitated the discussions and educated the family, linked them with counseling services, if necessary, and advocated for Flora and the children with the foster parents.

Some parents will not want their extended family and/or potential caregiver to know that they have HIV disease. Such parents should be encouraged to tell the future caregiver that they are asking them to consider taking the children because the parent has a potentially debilitating illness. If they not do so, the caregiver may not be making an informed decision. The caregiver may assume that the parent is asking "just in case something happens to me" and not understand that she (the caregiver) may be called upon to honor her commitment in the near future [Draimin 1995].

Negotiating with Potential Caregivers

Parents will want to clarify when the caregiver's plan should start, recommend how the children should be raised (for example education, religion), and talk about how they want the children to remember them.

> Joan gave guardianship of her children to her sister within a year of finding out that she had HIV. She wanted to know that provision had been made for her daughter and did not trust the legal system. Her daughter continued to live with her but stayed with the sister when her mother was hospitalized. Joan and her sister disagreed about when and how the custody transfer plan should take place. Joan wanted her daughter to live with her sister when she was very ill but wanted her daughter to visit if she wished to; the sister thought that when Joan had a severe illness or was terminal that all connections with her daughter should be severed. Joan thought family counseling would be helpful and hoped her sister would agree to attend.

Some parents who are considering the foster parent as a potential caregiver will decide to surrender their parental rights and arrange for adoption. In those instances, visiting and the openness of the relationship should be discussed.

> Andrea was living in a residential facility that did not allow children. She had thought long and hard about whether she could take care of her five children again. Her youngest child, a boy, had been in foster care since birth. She could see from her monthly visits that the child was well cared for. She decided that moving the now two-year-old child would not be in the child's best interests. She wondered if the foster mother would adopt her child. With the help of a social worker, Andrea educated herself about open adoption and prepared what she wanted to say to the foster mother. She talked at length with the child welfare worker to gain her support in arranging a meeting. The child welfare worker thought that the foster mother might be interested in adopting. At the meeting, Andrea and the foster mother agreed for Andrea's child to be adopted and

> negotiated certain conditions: the foster mother would always acknowledge that her son had "another" mother; the foster mother would let her son visit his siblings; and the foster mother would let Andrea continue to have occasional contact.

The worker had a critical role in making this arrangement. Prior to this meeting, Andrea had not had contact with the foster mother. The worker was the go-between initially for mother and foster mother. She also participated in the meeting, facilitating the discussion and mediating when necessary. If the foster mother was hesitant about meeting the biological mother, the worker would also have had to advocate for the biological mother. In some instances, family counseling is appropriate; the different players can sort out their differences and the children's voices can be heard. Workers may act as case managers and refer the family to appropriate services.

Making Legal Arrangements

The final task in HIV custody planning is formalizing the arrangement. Although this step seems simple and concrete, its finality requires emotional and practical preparation. Workers should be familiar with the different legal options in their state and make referrals to attorneys when families are ready.

Challenges to Custody Planning Within the Child Welfare System

The majority of women with HIV are low-income, minority women who live in inner-city environments [Hackl et al. 1997; Quinn 1993]. These women are among the least powerful and most oppressed in our society. Their mistrust of government and bureaucracy is based in history [Quinn 1993] and extends to child protective services. These women are already raising their children under difficult conditions, and perceive the child welfare system as a threat to one of the most important roles available to them—the role of parent. Each visit with the child and each contact by the worker are reminders of their deficiencies as parents. Women do not feel in control of the planning process if their children are out of their custody [Mason 1995] and, in reality, are often not consulted about service plans.

When parents are not included as partners in planning, they become adversaries. This stance of "me against the system" is not exclusive to HIV-infected parents. The adversarial relationship, however, may be aggravated when a worker's biases about HIV and the parent's sense of impatience clash. The parent works toward reunification as the only way to gain control over the children's lives and to be considered a "good" parent. After reunification, she feels she can think about custody planning in case of her death. This is acceptable—not every HIV-infected parent will plan for her children's future—but an opportunity is missed; a "door to service" has been closed that could benefit children, parents, and potential caregivers [Gruendel & Anderson 1995]. If child "welfare" services are provided in conjunction with child "protective" services, families can at least begin to tackle the activities in custody planning.

Because of the frequently adversarial nature of the client-worker relationship, the introduction of custody planning in case of the parent's death must be handled sensitively. Parents may perceive the worker as trying to get them to "give their children up" because they have AIDS. Introducing the idea in a nonthreatening manner, however, may be the most important role that a worker can take, because it opens the door to thinking and talking about future plans. A good relationship between the worker and the parent is the best basis, but not necessarily a prerequisite, for custody planning. One nonthreatening way of talking about planning is to generalize the approach. Mothers with AIDS often use chance as a reason to plan: "I could get hit by a bus tomorrow" is a common justification for planning for death. Using chance occurrences or accidents as a rationale removes the threat of HIV and generalizes planning to all parents who are concerned about their children.

Instead of focusing on a parent's deficits, strengths should be emphasized. Most parents care deeply about their children and want to make good decisions. Some parents may have voluntarily placed their children with the child welfare system because at the time they knew they could not care for them. Now they are being asked to make another important decision for their children. It helps them to know that making a plan is a difficult but crucial step toward the children's continued healthy life. Workers can give the parent control by discussing *all* of the options for each child. Though it is desirable to have some privacy for these talks, day-to-day opportunities to check in with a parent can reveal what he or she has been thinking. Court time, clinic time, and driving in the car are good opportunities to touch base. Written materials may reinforce the worker's message or allow parents to think and read about planning on their own time. Workbooks for planning are available through the Child Welfare League of America [Merkel-Holguin 1994] and local HIV/AIDS social service agencies.

Although parents may not follow through immediately, the worker, using the stratiegies above, will have planted the seed of an idea. If no progress develops during work with the parents, another helper may pick up the idea along the way. Workers often do not see grand results themselves but must trust that they are one of a series of helpers over time who will help a family make a custody plan. Mothers give the following advice to workers:

> Know where we are in the process of planning but do not push too hard if we are not ready. Raise the issue, back off if we resist, and bring it up again later. Stay on us about planning and support us but realize that you cannot make people do something if they are not ready. [Mason 1995]

Workers' Reactions to HIV and Death

Child welfare practice can be emotionally draining as workers deal with children and families in seemingly hopeless situations. Planning with HIV-infected mothers adds new dimensions to the work.

Custody planning with an HIV-infected mother is a constant reminder of one's own mortality. Watching other people struggle with their mortality raises one's own thoughts and feelings about death [Taylor-Brown 1995]. Workers must also come to terms with their own risk for HIV infection. Workers may see themselves in the clients they work with and back away in discomfort. Although most people are educated now about the behaviors that transmit HIV, practitioners, especially those new to the field, still face irrational fears of infection [Zayas & Romano 1994]. Confronted with their fears and prejudices, workers may forget that a parent's HIV disease, in and of itself, does not put a child at risk for abuse or neglect. HIV-infected mothers and fathers can be effective parents and they may be able to parent for years.

Some workers must bear the burden of holding secrets with the client family [Taylor-Brown 1995]. Perhaps a parent asks a worker not to tell the children or potential caregivers about the parent's HIV status; the worker disagrees with the choice but abides by the parent's decision. Workers may also have value conflicts with a client about pregnancy and abortion [Quinn 1993; Taylor-Brown 1995]. Simply having the information about a person's HIV status is a serious responsibility. Although people with HIV are living longer, parents who are clients will die. Workers feel their loss and their family's loss. The cumulative effect of loss and secrets can take a psychological and physical toll. Supervision, education, and other forms of agency support are essential to workers' good health. ◆

References

Blanche, S., Mayaux, M-J., & Veber, F. (1996). Separation between HIV-positive women and their children: The French prospective study, 1986 through 1993. *American Journal of Public Health, 86*, 376–91.

Bonuck, K. A. (1993). AIDS in families: Cultural, psychosocial, and functional impacts. *Social Work in Health Care, 18(2)*, 75–89.

Burton, L. M. (1992). Black grandparents rearing children of drug-addicted parents: Stressors, outcomes, and social service needs. *The Gerontologist, 12*, 744–751.

Cates, J. A., Graham, L. L., Boeglin, D., & Tielker, S. (1990). The effect of AIDS on the family system. *Families in Society 71*, 195–201.

Centers for Disease Control. (1996). *HIV/AIDS surveillance.* Atlanta, GA: U.S. Department of Health and Human Services.

Draimin, B. (1995). A second family? Placement and custody decisions. In S. Geballe, J. Gruendel, & W. Andiman (Eds.), *Forgotten children of the AIDS epidemic* (pp. 125–139). New Haven, CT: Yale University.

Draimin, B., Hudis, J., & Segura, J. (1992). *The mental health needs of well adolescents in families with AIDS.* New York: New York City Human Resources Administration, Division of AIDS Services.

Evans, M., Cohen, C., Shidlo, A., & deCaprariis, P. J. (1994). Counseling HIV-negative children of parents with HIV disease. *AIDS Patient Care, 8*(1), 16–19.

Florence, M.E., Lutzen, K., Alexius, B. (1994). Adaptation of heterosexually infected HIV-positive women: A Swedish pilot study. *Health Care for Women International, 15*, 265–273.

Gamble, I. (1993). *In whose care and custody.* New York: New York City Human Resources Administration, Division of AIDS services.

Gruendel, J. M., & Anderson, G. R. (1995). Building child- and family-responsive support systems. In S. Geballe, J. Gruendel, & W. Andiman (Eds.), *Forgotten children of the AIDS epidemic* (pp. 165–189). New Haven, CT: Yale University.

Hackl, K. L., Somlai, A. M., Kelly, J. A., & Kalichman, S. C. (1997). Women living with HIV/AIDS: The dual challenge of being a patient and caregiver. *Health and Social Work, 22*(1), 53–63.

Heller, T., & Factor, A. (1988). Permanency planning among black and white family caregivers of older adults with mental retardation. *Mental Retardation, 26*, 203–208.

Ickovics, J. R. & Rodin, J. (1992). Women and AIDS in the United States: Epidemiology, natural history, and mediating mechanisms. *Health Psychology, 11*, 1–16.

Levine, C. (1995). Today's challenges, tomorrow's dilemmas. In S. Geballe, J. Gruendel, & W. Andiman (Eds.), *Forgotten children of the AIDS epidemic* (pp. 190–204). New Haven, CT: Yale University.

LSC and Associates. (1994). *Report on the lives of Chicago women and children living with HIV infection.* Unpublished report submitted to Illinois Department of Children and Family Services, Chicago, IL.

Mason, S. (1995). *Mothers with AIDS: Planning for the future of their children* (unpublished doctoral dissertation, University of Illinois at Chicago).

McKelvy, L. (1993). The well children in AIDS families project: A hospital-based program. In C. Levine (Ed.), *A death in the family: Orphans of the HIV epidemic* (pp. 104–109). New York: United Hospital Fund of New York.

Merkel-Holguin, L. (1994). *Because you love them: A parent's planning guide.* Washington, DC: Child Welfare League of America, Inc.

Michaels, D., & Levine, C. (1992). Estimates of the number of motherless youth orphaned by AIDS in the United States. *Journal of the American Medical Association, 268,* 3456–3461.

Minkler, M., Driver, D., Roe, K., & Bedeian, K. (1993). Community interventions to support grandparent caregivers. *The Gerontologist,* 33, 807–811.

Monk, E. (1997, March). Personal communication. AIDS Project Coordinator, Illinois Department of Children and Family Services.

Quinn, S. C. (1993). AIDS and the African-American woman: The triple burden of race, class, and gender. *Health Education Quarterly, 20,* 305–320.

Smith, G. C., & Tobin, S. S. (1989) Permanency planning among older parents of adults with lifelong disabilities. *Journal of Gerontological Social Work, 14,* 35–59.

Tasker, M. (1992). *How can I tell you?* Bethesda, MD: Association for the Care of Children's Health.

Taylor-Brown, S. (1995). HIV-positive women: Finding a voice in the AIDS pandemic. In V. J. Lynch, G. A. Lloyd, & M. F. Fimbres (Eds.), *The changing face of AIDS: Implications for social work practice* (pp. 123–154). Westport, CT: Auburn.

Tiblier, K., Walker, G., & Rolland, J. (1989). Therapeutic issues when working with families of person with AIDS. In E. D. Macklin (Ed.), *AIDS and families* (pp. 88–128). New York: Haworth Press.

Wilson, P. A. (1995). HIV disease: Toward comprehensive services for families. In V. J. Lynch, G. A. Lloyd, & M. F. Fimbres (Eds.), *The changing face of AIDS: Implications for social work practice* (pp. 79–104). Westport, CT: Auburn.

Zayas, L. H., & Romano, K. (1994). Adolescents and parental death from AIDS. In B. O. Dane & C. Levine (Eds.), *AIDS and the new orphans: Coping with death* (pp. 59–76). Westport, CT: Auburn.

5 Improving Permanency Planning in Families with HIV Disease

Barbara H. Draimin, Ivy Gamble, Amy Shire, and Jan Hudis

This article describes two distinct service models developed for providing mental health and custody-planning services to families with advanced HIV disease or AIDS. Project Talk uses cognitive behavior techniques with groups of parents and their teenage children (ages 12 to 18). Project Care employs a psychoeducational approach to counseling mothers and children (ages 8 to 11) in their homes. While both models have a number of common characteristics, they also have unique strengths and limitations. Each is likely to play a role in providing services to a portion of the population facing the need to develop permanency plans for surviving children. Both models are being evaluated in separate longitudinal studies to assess the mental health outcomes of the children and the models' effectiveness in helping parents to plan for their futures.

Barbara H. Draimin, D.S.W., is Executive Director; Ivy Gamble, M.S.W., is Deputy Director; Amy Shire, M.P.H., is Program Manager; and Jan Hudis, M.P.H., M.P.A., is Research Manager, The Family Center, New York, NY.

Karen is a 36-year-old woman with AIDS. She has four children between 4 and 16 years of age and is pregnant. Because of her previous drug use, Karen is alienated from her mother and two sisters. She desperately wants to keep her children together and hopes that either her oldest child will assume that responsibility or that a volunteer who now cares for two of the children several days a month will ultimately be willing to take them all. Meanwhile, her children, aware of their mother's illness and uncertain about their own futures, are exhibiting a range of behavioral problems at home and in school.

There is no easy solution to Karen's custody concern, but she and her 16-year-old daughter are dealing candidly with some of its emotional and interpersonal issues through Project Talk, a group intervention developed at The Family Center of New York City. The Family Center was created in 1993 to help families with a terminally ill parent make custody plans for their children who survive the parent's death.

The Family Center's work is in response to the growing number of children who are likely to lose one or both of their parents to HIV disease. Little has been done to date to help affected families develop viable custody plans. Estimates of the number of children who will be orphaned by HIV disease, which has been defined for statistical purposes as losing their mothers, have risen steadily over the past few years. The first projections, based on fairly conservative assumptions, suggested that by the year 2000, the total number of motherless children and adolescents in the United States would exceed 80,000 and that 30,000 of these would be in New York City [Michaels & Levine 1992]. Updated estimates put the figure in New York City alone at about 50,000 by the end of 2001 [Working Committee 1996]. Of that number, nearly 90% will be African American or Latino.

Few systems of care exist to grapple with the complexities that surround illness disclosure and permanency planning. Researchers have found that more than half of the parents with AIDS die without having made a formal plan for the long-term care of their children [Draimin 1993]. Far fewer of those plans have actually been formalized legally. In many families, children have not even been told that a parent is living with AIDS, and little or nothing has been done to prepare them for their parent's death or to help them mourn afterwards. Eighty percent of the families are headed by mothers, 95% of whom are single parents [Draimin et al. 1992].

A needs assessment of healthy adolescents in families with AIDS identified four themes that characterize their experiences: (1) multiple losses, (2) isolation and lack of social supports, (3) destructive coping behaviors, and (4) problems identifying and maintaining new custodial placements [Gamble 1993; Hudis 1995]. This accords with studies showing that bereaved adolescents are more likely than their peers to be emotionally distressed, to experience behavior problems and impaired social relationships, and to engage in risk-taking practices [Weller & Weller 1991; Harris 1991; Dane & Miller 1992; Irwin & Millstein 1991]. Based on analogous situations, such as the impact of parental loss from cancer, it is apparent that "meeting the children's basic physical and emotional needs is a precondition to [their] mourning. If these needs are unmet, mourning may be inhibited because anxiety leads them to deny the loss" [Siegel & Gorey 1994].

Intervention is essential to lessen the risk for serious medical, behavioral, developmental, and learning problems, and to reduce the intergenerational patterns of risk-taking that may have led to the parents contracting HIV. Unless a supportive and stable environment is created to improve short-term and long-term mental health outcomes in orphaned children, a viable custody plan may not endure.

The Family Center developed two distinct service models to aid the formation of permanency plans. Project Talk, mentioned above, uses cognitive behavior techniques in group sessions with parents who have HIV disease and their teenage children, ages 12 to 18. The second model, Project Care, employs a psychoeducational approach to counseling infected mothers and their children in their homes. The decision to develop two different service models reflects a dual understanding. First, because the challenges posed by children likely to be orphaned by the HIV disease of their parents have only been recognized in the past few years, information about how best to serve this population is sparse, and pilot projects that take different approaches must be implemented and evaluated. Second, the needs of individuals and families differ, and more than one service approach is likely to be necessary. Both models are being evaluated in separate longitudinal studies.

Project Talk

Project Talk is an intensive, highly structured intervention funded by the National Institute of Mental Health. It is based on a cognitive behavior model: by increasing the coping skills of both the parent living with HIV and the adolescent children, Project Talk aims to minimize the long-term mental health consequences associated with the death of a parent that are often experienced by adolescents. Project Talk's premise is that parents need skills to maintain emotional self-control with their children, to manage the daily routines of the family, to decide when and how to disclose their illness, and to make custody arrangements for the children. For their part, adolescents need help to cope with parental demands, especially as the illness worsens; to maintain school performance and peer relationships despite family stressors; and to proceed through a bereavement process that enables them to deal with their loss.

The major themes, goals, activities, and skills to be targeted by Project Talk were identified in a series of focus groups that involved parents with AIDS who have teenage children and caseworkers in New York City's Division of AIDS Services. In addition, the literature on parental adjustment to other chronic and terminal illnesses was reviewed. Preliminary workshop sessions were pilot-tested, and the assessments and experiences of the first cohort helped to shape the design of the current intervention.

Families eligible for Project Talk are parents with advanced HIV disease who have at least one child between 12 and 18 years of age. The intervention has three parts, comprising eight to 16 fully scripted sessions, each lasting two hours (see figure 1). Three hundred six parents and 406 adolescents have participated in the project over four years. Transportation is provided from the urban neighborhoods where clients live to the central offices where the intervention is delivered. Food is provided and day care is available to families with young children who are not participating in Project Talk.

The objectives of Part 1, which has eight sessions for parents alone, are to help parents living with HIV disease recognize and cope with their own emotional responses to the diagnosis, to make and implement decisions about whether to disclose their illnesses, and to develop a future-oriented approach to coping with their children. Part 2 includes eight sessions, also for parents alone, that focus on aspects of parenting and on custody and estate planning. Eight concurrent sessions are scheduled for adolescents to deal with four major tasks: coping with parental illness, improving home life, avoiding risk behaviors, and planning for the future. Eight additional sessions in Part 2 bring together parents and adolescents, giving them an opportunity to confront their reactions to the illness and to talk about creating consistent, positive interactions at home. The eight sessions of Part 3 take place after the parent with HIV disease has died. The sessions are designed to help adolescents and their new caregivers move through the grieving process, participate in building a new, positive family unit, and obtain appropriate support from each other and from their peers.

To help facilitators achieve the project's objectives, a manual has been prepared that includes five components for each session: (1) a statement of goals, (2) the rationale, (3) a summary of the exercises and the time allowed for each one, (4) the materials needed, and (5) a scripted presentation of the facilitator's dialogue for each exercise in every session [Miller & Rotheram-Borus 1994]. Facilitators are trained to maintain the tight structure of each session and to be thoroughly familiar with the manual. They are encouraged, however, to present the exercises, which include role-playing, problem-solving, relaxation, and coping skills, in their own

FIGURE 1
The Project Talk Intervention

Part 1: Taking Care of Myself

Parent Curriculum

Session 1—Coping with my illness
Session 2—Coping with my fear
Session 3—Coping with anger
Session 4—Coping with sadness
Session 5—Coping with the meaning of my illness
Session 6—Coping with whether to tell
Session 7—Coping with telling others
Session 8—Coping with the future

Part 2: Illness

Parent Curriculum

Session 1—What are my children's needs?
Session 2—Who will take care of my children?
Session 3—What kind of arrangements can I make?
Session 4—How do I start my plan?
Session 5—How can I really listen to my children?
Session 6—How can I tell my children what I feel?
Session 7—How should I deal with problem behavior?

Adolescent Curriculum

Session 1—How do I make sense of my mother's illness?
Session 2—Should I tell someone my mother has AIDS?
Session 3—How can I deal with stigma?
Session 4—How do I deal with fear?
Session 5—How can I cope with feeling sad?
Session 6—What if I feel angry?
Session 7—What can I do about feeling angry?

Parent and Adolescent Curriculum

Session 8—How can we create a positive atmosphere at home?
Session 9—How can we resolve conflicts at home? (Part I)
Session 10—How can we resolve conflicts at home? (Part II)
Session 11—How can we work together on selecting a custodian?
Session 12—How can we deal with drugs and alcohol?
Session 13—How do I prevent pregnancy and fatherhood?

Parent Curriculum

Session 14—Where am I in making a custody plan?

Adolescent Curriculum

Session 14—How can we encourage safer sex?

Parent and Adolescent Curriculum

Session 15—How can mothers encourage safer sex?
Session 16—What is the mother's legacy and the youth's goals?

Part 3: Grieving

Adolescent and Guardian Curriculum

Session 1—What is grief?
Session 2—Helping with grief
Session 3—How can we create a strong family (appreciating and listening)?
Session 4—How can we create a strong family (expressing and solving)?
Session 5—How can I tolerate sadness?
Session 6—How can I deal with frightening situations?
Session 7—How can I handle feeling angry?
Session 8—What can we do about the future?

words. All of the facilitators have master's degrees and are supervised by a clinical psychologist.

To assess the effectiveness of Project Talk, the Family Center, in cooperation with the University of California at Los Angeles, began a four-year randomized clinical trial in 1993. A baseline interview is conducted with all participants at the time of enrollment, and mental health assessments of the adolescent participants and their parents continue every three months for two years. After a parent dies, the interviews continue with both the teenagers and their new caregivers. While evaluation data are not yet available, a preliminary assessment of the process suggests that the intervention can be delivered in a consistent manner.

Project Care

Project Care has been funded by the Ryan White Care ACT Title I and the Centers for Disease Control and Prevention since 1994. The project brings trained Family Specialists into the homes of clients with AIDS, who have at least one child, to help them create permanency plans for their minor children. A package of modules based on psychoeducational techniques guides the Family Specialists through focused conversations to lead ultimately to a legally formalized custody plan (see figure 2). Though the content of each session is somewhat more flexible than those of Project Talk, and the order of the sessions is adapted to the client's needs, the focus on permanency planning is always retained.

Part 1 of the Project Care intervention is delivered over a six-month period and focuses on disclosure and communication, custody-planning, and working with the new caregiver. Program components are delivered in eight two-hour sessions by Family Specialists who are bachelor's- and master's-level social workers with at least two years experience working with families and two years experience with people with AIDS. The Family Specialists also meet with and assess the children and the proposed caregiver,

Figure 2
Project Care Modules—Part 1

Core Program—Parent	Optional Services—Parent
Considering clinical trials	A primer on healthy eating
Counseling for pregnant women	Advance directives
Talking to others about illness	Relaxation and stress reduction
Talking to a child about the child's illness	Creating a memory bank
How are your children doing?	
Permanency planning options	
Choosing a future caregiver	
Joint visit with the future caregiver and parent	
Going to court	

Core Program—Caregivers	
Services and entitlements for children and new families	Grief and loss
Family adjustment	Looking to the future

but the focus remains on the ill parent and on making custody arrangements.

In addition to the in-home services provided by Family Specialists, three staff members review each case and become directly involved in providing services. Their participation is based on the belief that a permanency plan can succeed only if the tools are provided for interfacing with three separate systems—psychosocial services, the legal system, and entitlement programs. Toward that goal, a social worker visits many families to assess the children's mental health, provide short-term counseling, and make referrals for therapy, if necessary. Three full-time staff lawyers are available to make home visits where they provide legal assistance, including explaining legal options, drawing up a will or custody petitions, arranging standby guardianship, and initiating adoption proceedings. The third member of the support team is a benefits and housing specialist who provides consultation about financial, housing, health care, and other concrete services and entitlement programs. All Project Care providers meet weekly with a social work coordinator who provides supervision and oversight. Linkages to community resources are another important activity of Project Care; they are designed to avoid service duplication while ensuring that clients receive the full package of services they need.

Not all clients opt to use all of the modules. Instead, parents choose from a list of topics and indicate the preferred sequence so that the intervention deals first with client-identified needs. The objective is to build trust so that the mother becomes receptive to dealing with issues that are increasingly more challenging, both emotionally and logistically, such as disclosure and custody planning.

Disclosure and Communication

Disclosure is dealt with on a continuum that spans not disclosing anything, to saying one is ill, or has a serious illness, or has HIV, or has AIDS, or may die. The disclosure component is based on the premise that disclosure of parental illness (not necessarily HIV) to the children and the future caregiver is optimal for open communication, to prepare the child for the parent's death, and to develop a custody plan. Worker experience has shown that parents who do not want to disclose their illness to older children or future caregivers may place the viability of the plan in jeopardy. The choice to disclose illness or HIV to any party remains with the parent, however, and is always respected by the worker.

There are many steps in examining disclosure: assessing the extent of disclosure to family members and determining who in the family knows the severity of the mother's illness; identifying impediments to disclosure, such as stigmatization and discrimination; discussing the burdens of secrecy and disclosure; building trust with the mother by encouraging her to control the decision regarding who is told the diagnosis; helping the mother determine the desired level of disclosure and discussing family reactions to disclosure; assessing the extent of existing maternal and child social supports and introducing strategies to enhance support; and helping the mother accept the importance of preparing the children for the mother's death and of planning for their future.

Family Specialists respect and honor the parent's decision about whether, what, and to whom to disclose illness and/or HIV status.

Custody and Planning

The custody component helps parents take concrete steps to prepare for their children's future. The aims are to help parents identify and designate a new caregiver for each child; to establish a viable custody plan for each child; to assess the child's knowledge about the illness (including knowledge of the AIDS diagnosis) and the level of associated behavioral and emotional problems; and to assess the child's feelings about the designated new caregiver. The intervenor facilitates open communication and helps the child prepare for the parent's death while adhering to parental wishes in relation to disclosing the AIDS diagnosis.

Working with the New Caregiver

The new caregiver component of the intervention begins as soon as is practical and aims to assure that the assigned caregiver has agreed to take legal custody of the children after the parent's death. Other goals involve conducting a needs assessment that anticipates problems after placement and begins to provide solutions; assessing eligibility of the new caregiver for social services now and in the future and expediting the necessary applications; evaluating the caregiver's support system and improving aspects that are inadequate; and providing support and referral to the new caregiver concerning child rearing and strategies for helping bereaved children.

After Part 1 is completed, the Family Specialist maintains monthly telephone contact with the family and the new caregiver to assure that the custody plan remains viable, to confirm the client's address, and to stay current with the family's health status. Part 2 of Project Care begins after the parent's death and focuses on the new family's adjustment. This phase is delivered in four two-hour sessions and emphasizes the needs of the caregiver and the children in adjusting to a new family.

New Family Adjustment

This component is designed to assist the new family during the transition period, when the custody plan is most at risk, and to provide children and their caregivers with regular access to the Family Specialist. Part of the effort is a supportive intervention to assist the child and the caregiver through the grief process. Specifically, the intervenor helps families recognize the different dimensions of bereavement, and assists caregivers to recognize the wide variety of bereavement reactions that may emerge, to understand that children mourn differently than adults, and to identify when bereavement has become more complicated and more intensive and specialized intervention is called for. In addition, the intervenor helps the caregiver to access community services so that the opportunity to provide sustained care is protected; helps families arrange transportation and child care, as necessary, and serves as an escort; provides follow-up to determine whether families have accessed referrals; helps the child identify people who can provide support and intervene with the caregiver to assure that the child has opportunities to express painful or conflicting emotions and fantasies; focuses the caregiver's attention on the importance of consistency, predictability, and security to children, and helps the caregiver to develop dependable routines for the children; and helps mobilize natural supports.

The evaluation component of Project Care is supported by grants from the Centers for Disease Control and Prevention as well as the National Institute of Mental Health. It describes the permanency planning process in families with AIDS and identifies both the risks and the protective factors that influence the adjustment of children experiencing the death of a parent from AIDS.

Comparing the Models

Project Talk and Project Care are both longitudinal interventions that are being carefully evaluated, the former through a randomized trial and the latter through a descriptive study. They share a number of key characteristics. The populations served are quite similar—primarily families of African American and Latino descent who are Medicaid-eligible clients of New York City's Department of Social Services. Eighty percent of the adult clients are mothers and are typically the exclusive caregiver in the family.

Because the crisis of an AIDS diagnosis reverberates throughout a family, the interventions are predicated on the belief that services should be targeted at both the family unit and the individuals within that unit. In general, both projects recognize the need to assess the availability of resources known to help child adjustment and, where necessary, to enhance them, as well as to find ways to avoid the unnecessary pile-up of additional stressors and risk factors. Both projects have as their underlying objective the development of a viable permanency plan that will lead to a reasonable degree of stability for the surviving children.

For many clients, HIV disease carries a heavy stigma among family members and within the community. The group setting of Project Talk reduces isolation while fostering supportive connections. Interactions with peers facing similar challenges not only reduce feelings of being alone but may sharpen the relevance of, and lend credibility to, the issues being discussed and the lessons learned. In particular, parents may be able to learn skills of conflict resolution most effectively by working together, while adolescents may find valuable outlets for expressing their emotional conflicts among peers.

Although a formal cost analysis has not been undertaken, the group sessions of Project Talk are likely to be more expensive than in-home counseling because substantial transportation, food, and day care costs are incurred. In addition, clients are less likely to appear for group sessions in another neighborhood than to be home as scheduled to receive the individual counseling services offered through Project Care.

Another limitation of the group approach concerns confidentiality. Although the rule that nothing said within the group is to be shared with others is repeatedly emphasized, it takes time for clients to develop sufficient trust with one another to be fully candid. A further complication related to privacy and confidentiality is that participation in Project Talk requires that parents must have told their adolescent children that they have HIV, which excludes a portion of the otherwise eligible population.

The in-home counseling strategy used by Project Care has its own strengths and limitations. On the positive side, it allows for a maximum level of individual attention and makes it difficult for a client to remain quiet or hidden, as can occur in group settings. Additionally, the logistics of providing services are often easier to arrange and many families appreciate professionals making the effort to visit their home. Project Care also minimizes confidentiality concerns, although Family Specialists must take special care to recognize and respect the level of disclosure that has already occurred within the family. Special challenges to in-home service provision include the lack of opportunity for peer support and the difficulty of establishing and monitoring quality control standards for service delivery.

A number of thematic threads run through Project Talk and Project Care. Recruiting families into each intervention has been a continual challenge. This is explained, to some degree, by the readiness to plan within the household, as well as the inner turmoil families experience, such as ongoing substance use, financial pressures, housing insecurities, emotional stress, and behavioral problems among the children, as well as by the privacy matters already mentioned.

Disclosure remains a highly sensitive consideration not only at the time of enrollment but throughout the intervention. Practitioners must recognize how extraordinarily difficult disclosure can be for clients and must acknowledge and respect clients' feelings about it. At the same time, clients must be guided toward a recognition of the value of illness disclosure as a necessary step in completing permanency planning. Disparities often appear between what parents believe their children know and what the children actually understand; and these differences have to be reconciled if movement is to go on. Research and evaluation must refine the tools that at once facilitate disclosure and provide necessary support to all parties.

The relationship between the future caregiver and the parents also demands great delicacy. Many parents are highly invested in their parental role and indeed may say that a sense of responsibility for their children helps keep them alive, though the illness itself often makes it difficult for them to fulfill parenting obligations. Discussion about permanency planning compels parents to confront the realities of illness and to acknowledge the eventual possibility of surrendering the care of their children to others. This may foster resentment toward the caregiver, as well as great sadness, yet parents are likely to feel a tremendous sense of relief when adequate custody arrangements are put in place. These mixed and contradictory emotions create challenges for caregivers trying to assess their own role within the family while the parent remains alive.

One of the most painful limitations of both the Project Talk and Project Care initiatives is the necessity of bringing client wishes and dreams into alignment with the realities of what is possible. For both clients and providers, there is often a degree of wishful thinking about caregiving options. In truth, a perfect plan seldom exists and most arrangements are potentially vulnerable. Acknowledging the constraints and emphasizing the importance of reinforcing or discarding shaky plans is perhaps the most constructive way of dealing with the boundaries of what is possible.

Conclusion

There is no evidence to suggest that either Project Talk or Project Care is in any way a superior model. To the contrary, each has distinctive advantages and disadvantages and each may well be suitable to a particular subset of the population of families with HIV disease. Other approaches, such as residential programs and buddy programs, may also be appropriate for some families; pilot projects should be developed to learn more about them. Only by implementing and evaluating multiple models for providing services to families can funders and practitioners expect to identify the most suitable opportunities for building a stable future for the children orphaned by HIV disease. ◆

References

Dane, B. & Miller, S. (1992). AIDS: *Intervening with hidden grievers*. Westport, CT: Auburn House.

Draimin, B., Hudis, J., & Segura, J. (1992). *The mental health needs of well adolescents in families with AIDS*. New York: Human Resources Administration, Division of AIDS Services.

Draimin, B. (1993). Adolescents in families with AIDS: Growing up with loss. In C. Levine (Ed.), *A death in the family: Orphans of the HIV Epidemic* (pp. 13–23). New York: United Hospital Fund.

Gamble, I. (1993). *In whose care and custody: Placement and policies for children whose parents die of AIDS*. New York: The Family Center & The Orphan Project.

Harris, E. (1991). Adolescent bereavement following the death of a parent: An exploratory study. *Child Psychiatry and Human Development, 21*, 267–281.

Hudis, J. (1995). Adolescents in families with AIDS. In S. Geballe, J. Gruendel, & W. Andiman (Eds.), *The mental health needs of well adolescents in families with AIDS* (pp. 83–94). New Haven, CT: Yale University Press.

Irwin, C., & Millstein, S. (1991). Risk-taking behaviors during adolescence. In R. M. Lerner, A. C. Peterson, & J. Brooks-Gunn (Eds.), *Encyclopedia of adolescence* (pp. 934–943). New York: Garland.

Michaels, D., & Levine, C. (1992). Estimates of the number of motherless youth orphaned by AIDS in the United States. *Journal of the American Medical Association, 268*, 3456–61.

Miller, S., & Rotheram-Borus, M. J. (1994). Project T.A.L.C.: Teens and parents learning to communicate. Los Angeles: University of California.

Siegel, K., & Gorey, E. (1994). Childhood bereavement in AIDS orphans. *Journal of Developmental and Behavioral Pediatrics, 15*, 58–62.

Weller, E., & Weller, R. (1991). Grief. In M. Lewis (Ed.), *Child and adolescent psychiatry: A comprehensive textbook* (pp. 389–94). Baltimore: William and Wilkins.

Working Committee on HIV, Children, and Families. (1996). *Families in crisis*. New York: Federation of Protestant Welfare Agencies.

6 Correlates and Distribution of HIV Risk Behaviors Among Homeless Youths in New York City: Implications for Prevention and Policy

Michael C. Clatts, W. Rees Davis, J. L. Sotheran, and Aylin Atillasoy

Homeless youths are at high risk for poor health outcomes, including repeated exposure to STDs and high rates of unplanned pregnancies, untreated TB, HIV infection, and accelerated immune dysfunction associated with AIDS. This article examines the nature and distribution of HIV-risk behavior in a broad, street-based sample of homeless and runaway youths in New York City (*N* = 929). Although street youths in general are shown at high risk, the highest risks nest within older age segments of the male street youth population. Paradoxically, these youths are least likely to be in contact with prevention services. The data demonstrate the need to reconsider the use of chronological age as a determinant for service eligibility and to reconfigure funding streams so as to more effectively and consistently target older and more vulnerable youths.

Michael C. Clatts, Ph.D., is Principal Investigator; W. Rees Davis, Ph.D., is Co-Investigator; J.L. Sotheran, Ph.D., is Co-Investigator; and Aylin Atillasoy, Ph.D, is Co-Investigator; Youth at Risk Project, Institute for AIDS Research, National Development Research Institutes, Inc., New York, NY. The Youth at Risk Project was established as a

An estimated two million youths are homeless in the U.S.; some 200,000 of these youths live as permanent residents of the streets [U.S. Department of Health and Human Services 1986]. In New York City, this population is estimated to be as high as 20,000 youths [Schaffer & Caton 1984]. Some of these youths are transitionally homeless, having left home for a brief period of time [Adams et al. 1985; Dunford 1976]. Many others, however, have gone to the streets because they are unwelcome at home. Youths frequently cite conflict over sexual identity as a factor in their homelessness. Other youths become homeless because their families have become homeless or simply because their families are economically unable to continue to care for them [Benker et al. 1990; Clatts et al. 1997; Gunn 1988; Kufeldt & Nimmo 1987; Pries & Silbert 1991]. Service providers working with this population report that as many as two-thirds have "discharged" themselves from out-of-home care—often for many of the same reasons that youths not in care leave home, including physical and sexual abuse, conflict over sexual identity, and breakdown of the family as a viable socioeconomic unit.

Whatever the genesis of their move to the streets, it is clear that most of these youths enter street life at an age at which they are ill prepared to manage the social and economic tasks associated with becoming healthy, functioning adults. Many remain homeless for prolonged periods of time and face overwhelming obstacles in any effort to leave street life [Clatts et al. 1995; Clatts et al. in press]. Limited education, lack of marketable job skills,

collaborative effort of the National Development and Research Institutes, Inc., Victims Services Agency, the Hetrick-Martin Institute, the Community Health Project, the Center for Children and Families, and the AIDS and Adolescence Network of New York. Data are derived from studies funded by the Centers for Disease Control (grant #U62/CCU207192-01), the National Institute on Drug Abuse (grant #271–90–8402), and the American Foundation for AIDS Research (grant #00214–16–RG). The authors acknowledge the support of Marie Bresnahan, Richard Haymes, Frances Kunreuther, Helene Lauffer, Teri Lewis, John Santelli, Edith Springer, Mary Washburn, and John Wright. The views presented in this article are those of the authors and do not necessarily represent the position of any of the aforementioned institutions or individuals.

and the generalized emotional and cognitive instability associated with homelessness itself contribute to these youths' dependency on "the street economy" (e.g., sex trade, panhandling, drug dealing) as the primary source for money with which to meet their basic needs for food, clothing, and shelter [Clatts & Davis 1993; Kipke et al. 1995; Yates et al. 1988]. The constellation of sex and drug risk behaviors, together with the chronic and progressively debilitating exposure to the street environment itself, creates exceptional vulnerability to a number of poor health outcomes—including sexually transmitted diseases, hepatitis, tuberculosis, enteric parasites, bronchial infections, asthma, pneumonia, conjunctivitis, depression, and malnutrition—and to an alarming rate of HIV infection.

Available data on the incidence of HIV infection among these youths are scarce but suggest that a substantial number have already been exposed to HIV [D'Angelo et al. 1991; Futterman et al. 1993]. For example, a double-blind 1990 study conducted in a shelter for homeless youths indicated an overall HIV seroprevalence of over 5% [Stricof et al. 1991]. Prevalence was even higher among older male youths, of whom 10% were seropositive. While alarming in their own right, these estimates probably significantly underestimate actual levels of infection since the particular institutional context in which they were collected was unlikely to have included representative proportions of gay, lesbian, or bisexual youths. These latter populations might be expected to evidence higher seroprevalence, reflecting their multiple risks for infection and the high background seroprevalence of the populations with whom they interact in the context of both high-risk sexual behavior and high-risk drug use [Clatts et al. 1994]. Clearly, this is a population that is at exceptionally high risk for AIDS and a number of other poor health outcomes.

This article examines the prevalence of risk behaviors associated with HIV/AIDS in a broad, street-based sample of homeless and runaway youths in New York City, and the distribution of risk behaviors and their correlation with age. The authors consider problematic the assumption that chronological age is an appropriate marker for structuring prevention services oriented to high-risk youth populations.

Study Design and Methods

Data were collected as part of a CDC-funded evaluation of AIDS outreach and prevention services. Four rounds of cross-sectional surveys were conducted among youths between the ages of 12 and 23 who were homeless and/or dependent upon the street economy ($N = 929$). Additional longitudinal data were collected as part of ethnographic studies funded by the National Institute on Drug Abuse and the American Foundation for AIDS Research ($N = 30$). Youths were contacted on the streets using a time-by-location sampling plan that systematically canvassed designated sampling locations which formative ethnographic research had identified as areas in which high concentrations of these youths could be found [Clatts et al. 1995]. Eligibility was restricted to youths who had spent at least one night in the past year sleeping on the streets, or in subways, abandoned buildings, or homeless shelters, and/or to youths who, regardless of their housing status, depended on the street economy (e.g., panhandling, stealing, drug distribution, prostitution) as the primary means by which they acquired money for food and shelter. In tandem with the street-based survey interviews, a subsample of youths was recruited for participation in a longitudinal ethnographic study concerned with documenting the process by which youths enter the street economy and how they come to adopt particular roles within it, especially roles associated with increased risk for HIV infection.

The ethnographic data suggested that exposure to risk and chronic involvement in risk behavior increased as youths grew older and more deeply entrenched in the street economy [Clatts et al. in press]. Paradoxically, older youths also appeared likely to be estranged from prevention services. To examine the generalizability of these patterns in a broader sample of the street youth population, the cross-sectional sample was disaggregated into two-year age groups. Chi-square analyses were used to compare both HIV risk behaviors and contact with HIV prevention services among age groups.

Demographic and Behavioral Profile

The majority (74%) of the youths in the sample were male [Clatts & Davis 1993]. Two-thirds identified as ethnic minorities, primarily African American (29%) or Hispanic (30%). One-third (35%) self-identified as gay, lesbian, or bisexual. Over two-thirds (69%) were homeless at the time of the interview—living on the streets and sleeping in parks, subways, bus stations, and abandoned buildings. Of the youths who were homeless at the time of the interview, over two-thirds (67%) had been on the streets for more than one year.

Although more than one-quarter of the sample had held some kind of legal job in the past six months, most were also engaged in a number of illegal or quasi-legal activities within the street economy. Over a third (37%) panhandled. Nearly one-quarter (24%) were involved in some form of illegal drug distribution. One-quarter (25%) acknowledged being involved in prostitution, although this figure probably significantly underrepresents the number who are engaged in informal sexual transactions for food, shelter, or drugs that may not be defined as prostitution. Well over a third (38%) reported having multiple episodes of unprotected sex with different partners. Nearly a third (28%) had been diagnosed with a sexually transmitted disease, although this probably underrepresents the actual rate of STD infection in this population, as STDs in this population often go unrecognized and untreated.

Among the youths surveyed, there was a high prevalence of both lifetime and current use of a wide range of illegal drugs. Over two-thirds (68%) had used some type of hard drugs (other than alcohol and marijuana). Over half had used cocaine (53%), a third had used amphetamines (32%), over a third had used crack (36%), over a third had used heroin (38%), and over half had used psychedelics such as LSD (51%). Nearly a third (30%) had injected drugs at some time in their life and roughly half of these had shared drug injection paraphernalia (including syringes, cottons, and cookers). One in five were unable to estimate their risk for HIV infection. Of those who did venture an estimation of risk, two-thirds believed that they were "likely" or "very likely" to "get AIDS." Only about one-fifth (22%) of the sample had ever been contacted by street outreach and prevention services. Despite high levels of drug involvement, less than one-quarter (24%) had ever been in drug treatment.

Age Distribution of Risk

In examining risk behaviors within the sample with particular attention to age distribution, the proportion having both lifetime (ever) and current (last 30 days) sexual risk is significantly higher in older age groups (ages 19 to 23)—reaching the highest levels in the oldest age group (ages 22 to 23 years). For example, the proportions of youths having ever had unprotected sex with multiple partners ($p < .001$) and having ever had unprotected sex with a main partner ($p < .05$) are both significantly higher among youths aged 22 to 23 years. Similarly, these youths are significantly more likely to be currently involved in commercial sex work ($p < .001$)—trading sex for food, shelter, money, and/or drugs. These patterns are consistent with self-reported STDs, with the older youths being significantly more likely to have had an STD ($p < .001$). Youths aged 22 to 23 years are also significantly more likely to have had lifetime involvement in drug injection ($p < .001$) and more likely to be currently (in the preceding 30 days) engaged in drug injection ($p < .01$). A similar pattern is evident in reported use of crack-cocaine—a drug that is closely tied to involvement in street prostitution where it is used to stay awake and alert, to stave off hunger, and to self-medicate negative feelings associated with sexual work. Older youths are significantly more likely to have ever used crack ($p < .001$) as well as to be current users of crack ($p < .001$).

The high prevalence of both sexual risk and injection risk in the same population—and often within the same individuals—is of particular concern because these two risk behaviors account for such a large proportion of AIDS cases in New York City. For example, in the cumulative adult male AIDS cases in New York City from 1981 through 1996 (78% of the total cases), 44% are attributed to sex with men, 42% to injection drug use, and 4% to sex with a male injection drug user [New York City Department of Health 1996]. That youths in general are not exempt from these risks is shown by their contribution to the diagnosed AIDS cases among adolescents and young adults; these cases make up approximately 15% of the total cumulative cases and increasingly account for a larger share of newly reported cases [New York City Department of Health 1996]. Thus, even in the absence of definitive seroprevalence data specific to the street youth population, the large number of diagnosed AIDS cases in New York City that involve men who have sex with men and drug injectors suggests that homeless youths are particularly vulnerable because such a high proportion of them—compared with the general adolescent and young adult population—engage in one or both of these risk behaviors with one or both of these two populations with high background seroprevalence.

Unfortunately, although the behavioral data demonstrate that older street youths are at significantly greater risk for HIV, they are at the same time the least likely to be contacted by outreach and prevention services or to use these services [Clatts & Davis 1996a]. The principal gateway into the service delivery system for this population is through street outreach programs. Only about one-fifth of the total sample, however, had contact with any kind of street-based prevention or care services within the 30 days prior to their interview, reflecting the great dearth of resources available for these services relative to the acute needs of this population as a whole. In stratifying the sample along the dimension of age, the proportion that had a recent contact with prevention services significantly declines in the older age groups within the sample ($p < .01$), indicative of the fact that as youths become older, they are less likely to be in contact with prevention services, including street outreach. Thus, although contact with street outreach services was shown to significantly increase the utilization of prevention services by youths in the sample as a whole [Clatts & Davis 1996b]—including local youth-oriented drop-in centers, housing services, drug treatment, general health services, STD screening and treatment, and HIV testing and counseling—the protective effects of these services are not extended to older street youths.

The correlation between age and estrangement from services is of particular concern for the older segment of the street youths population. Due to time delays between exposure and the onset of symptoms, it is the older segments of the street youth population who are most likely to evidence HIV-related illnesses. The fact that this particular part of the street youth population is the least likely to be in contact with AIDS care services raises both clinical and policy concerns. Clinically, it suggests that many of these youths will not receive services until they are in end-stage disease—a point at which these youths are generally much more difficult to manage and much more expensive to care for. Moreover, it suggests that relatively few street youths are likely to benefit from recent advances in HIV treatment [Clatts et al. 1997] because they are unlikely to be able to access the kinds of support services needed both to obtain treatment and to support the compliance burden. Finally, estrangement from services among these older youths is also alarming in terms of the lost opportunity to foster secondary prevention, a circumstance that is likely to result in increased new HIV infections since these youths are most likely to be acutely dependent upon street prostitution.

Discussion

As described earlier, the statistical data were collected as part of a larger, multicity study that employed a cross-sectional design. Consequently, inferences about correlations between risk behaviors and age are based upon stratification of the sample across two-year age groups, rather than by examining risk behavior in the same individual over time (an approach that was employed in the smaller ethnographic subsample). The statistical data must, therefore, be approached with some caution, particularly in the context of a population such as this about which relatively little is known. An additional limitation of these data stems from the fact that the instrument employed in the study did not include questions about when youths first entered the street economy or when they had first engaged in a particular risk behavior. Consequently, at the level of the individual, it is impossible to disentangle chronological age and onset of risk behavior, and therefore to examine the question of age in relation to "person-years at risk." Moreover, within the confines of this study, it was not possible to formally measure developmental delay.

It is noteworthy, however, that parallel ethnographic evidence collected from a subsample in which a longitudinal design was employed provides us with a reasonable basis for making inferences about the relationship between age and risk behavior in this population. These patterns have substantially informed the interpretation of statistical data that has been presented here. In the ethnographic subsample, young, relatively inexperienced youths not yet knowledgeable enough about the street economy were found to have limited "mobility" in terms of their roles and economic opportunities within the street economy. The vast majority report entry into the street economy in the context of survival sex and using daily sex work as the principal means of acquiring money for that day's food and shelter.

The emotional degradation that is typical of this kind of sexual exploitation becomes progressively debilitating over time, and the ethnographic interviews are filled with descriptions of self-hate, self-blame, and feelings of self-destruction. As the cumulative effects of these emotions become more terrifying and more overwhelming, youths respond with increased self-medication through the use of street drugs, particularly stimulant drugs such as crack cocaine. The proportion of money used to support drug use draws an increasingly larger share of youths' "incomes," soon overtaking other needs such as food, clothing, and shelter, and perpetuating youths' involvement in, and dependence upon, the sex-for-drugs cycle of exchange. As the inherent limits of income that are achievable from the sex trade are reached, or during periods in which usual street "hustles" are unproductive, youths' economic strategies become more desperate—selling sex for less money, engaging in unprotected sex in exchange for higher rewards, and turning to alternative roles in the street economy (notably within drug distribution) that generally involve greater levels of interpersonal violence.

Consistent with the findings evidenced in the survey, ethnographic research in the street environments in which these youths participate indicates that older youths are more heavily drug dependent, are routinely involved in drug-related violence (notably violent sex work), and are more likely to be in acute and chronic emotional distress—all of which might be expected to be correlated with increased social alienation, including estrangement from services. While these patterns can, in some respects, be seen to stem from factors within the youths themselves, these data suggest that they are also, at least in part, a function of the way in which the service delivery system itself is structured. The apparent contradiction between the preponderance of risk behavior being situated in older age groups (youth who are at the same time least likely to be engaged in and by prevention services) is a direct consequence of service priorities and resource allocations that favor younger segments of the street youth population. These policies create functional obstacles to accessing youth-oriented services as chronological (i.e., legal) adult age is achieved, although this is precisely the segment that evidences the highest levels of risk, and despite the fact that there is often a poor clinical "fit" between legalistic definitions of adolescence (based on chronological age) and the widespread developmental delays that are evidenced in this population as a result of chronic violence and victimization.

The rationale for the existing funding structure is that youths can be moved on to adult services, a proposition that is belied by these data, which clearly show that older youths are least likely to access any type of prevention services. In reality, as these youths are increasingly the victims of the rationing of youth-oriented services, they are effectively abandoned to the vagaries of the streets where they are unlikely to reappear in surveillance data until they enter the criminal system for having committed a violent crime or are seen in a hospital emergency room with acute disease. Both are negative outcomes, in terms of pain and suffering for the individual as well as in terms of costs to the community.

The data presented here suggest that there is a need to rethink the way in which prevention services for the homeless are structured, particularly assumptions about different age groups within the overall homeless population. This requires the development of effective program models for different groups within the street-involved youth population as well as changes in funding streams with which to support these targeted services. The need for these changes has become all the more evident as a growing number of street youths have become infected with HIV and face AIDS-related illness. The vast majority of the street youths evidencing AIDS-related health problems are in their early twenties, the very age group to which youth service providers are being forced to deny services because of age-mandates of prevailing funding structures.

Conclusion

Adolescence is a complex period of profound physical, psychological, and social transitions. When the exigencies of street life are added to the equation, the picture becomes even more complex. Street youths are particularly difficult to engage for service delivery, as the stress and emotional trauma that characterize their everyday lives render them distrustful of existing mainstream service delivery systems and they often lack the requisite skills to access the system. Although street outreach has been recognized as an effective engagement strategy, and has been shown to have particular efficacy in connecting and retaining street youths in critical health promotion services [Clatts & Davis 1996b], the resources to support these programs are in dire jeopardy. In part, at least, the funding crisis is a function of contemporary fiscal policies that promote the consolidation of community-based prevention services—policies whose net effect is the elimination of many targeted services for specialized populations, including particular segments of the high-risk youth population who are at exceptional risk for HIV infection and AIDS-related illnesses. ◆

References

Adams, G. R., Gullotta, T., & Clancy, M. (1985). Homeless adolescents: A descriptive study of similarities and differences between runaways and throwaways. *Adolescence, 20,* 715–724.

Benker, K., Boone, M., & Dehavenon, A. (1990). *The tyranny of indifference: A study of hunger, homelessness, poor health, and family dismemberment in 1,325 New York City households with children, 1989–1990.* New York: The Action Research Project on Hunger, Homelessness and Family Health.

Clatts, M. C., Hillman, D. J., Atillasoy, A., & Davis, W.R. (in press). Lives in the balance: An ethnographic profile of homeless youth in New York City. In J. Bluestein & C. Levine (Eds.), *Medical decision-making for adolescents who are alone.*

Clatts, M. C., Sotheran, J. L., Lewis, T. L., Galatowitsch, P., & Alpert, E. (1997, July). *Needs assessment: Services and housing for New York City's homeless street youth with HIV/AIDS. Final Report.* Submitted to the Mayor's Office for AIDS Policy Coordination.

Clatts, M. C., & Davis, W. R. (1996a). *Correlates of homelessness among street youth in NYC: Implications for targeting AIDS prevention services.* Paper presented at the 11th International Conference on AIDS, Vancouver, British Columbia.

Clatts, M. C., & Davis, W. R. (1996b). *Enhancing the protective effects of AIDS outreach programs for homeless youth: A community-based model for integrating health and human services.* Paper presented at the 124th Annual Meeting of the American Public Health Association, New York.

Clatts, M. C., & Davis, W. R. (1993). *A demographic and behavioral profile of homeless youth in New York City: Implications for AIDS outreach and prevention.* Paper presented at the annual meeting of the American Public Health Association, San Francisco, California.

Clatts, M. C., Davis, W. R., & Atillasoy, A. (1995). Hitting a moving target: The use of ethnographic methods in the evaluation of AIDS outreach programs for homeless youth in NYC. *Qualitative Methods in Drug Abuse and HIV Research. NIDA Research Monograph* 157, 117–135.

Clatts, M. C., Davis, W. R., & Sotheran, J. L. (1994). *At the cross-roads of HIV infection: A demographic and behavioral profile of street youth in NYC*. Paper presented at the Second Symposium on Drugs, Sex, and AIDS: Prevention Research 1995-2000, Flagstaff, Arizona.

D'Angelo, L. J., Getson, P. R., Luban, N. L., & Gayle, H. D. (1991). Human immunodeficiency virus infection in urban adolescents: Can we predict who is at risk? *Pediatrics, 88*, 982–986.

Dunford, F., & Brennan, T. (1976). A taxonomy of runaway youth. *Social Services Review*, 50, 457–470.

Futterman, D., Hein, K., Reuben, N., Dell, R., & Schaffer, N. (1993). Human immunodeficiency virus-infected adolescents: The first 50 patients in a New York City program. *Pediatrics, 91*, 730–735.

Gunn, B. (1988). *Results of the study of street youths and runaways*. New York: Office of the Mayor.

Kipke, M. C., O'Connor, S., Palmer, R., & MacKenzie, R. (1995). Street youth in Los Angeles: Profile of a group at high risk for human immunodeficiency virus infection. *Archives of Pediatric and Adolescent Medicine, 149*(5), 513–519.

Kufeldt, K., & Nimmo, M. (1987). Youth on the street: Abuse and neglect in the eighties. *Child Abuse and Neglect, 11*, 531–43.

New York City Department of Health. (1996). AIDS surveillance update (Third Quarter/October).

Pries, S. & Silbert, J. (1991). *On their own: Runaway and homeless youth and programs that serve them*. Washington, DC: Georgetown University Child Development Center.

Schaffer, D., & Caton, S. (1984). *Runaway and homeless youth in New York City*. New York: Ittelson Foundation.

Stricof, R., Kennedy, J., Natell, T., Weisfuse, I., & Novick, L. (1991). HIV seroprevalence in a facility for runaway and homeless adolescents. *American Journal of Public Health, 81*, (supplement), 50–53.

United States Department of Health and Human Services (1986). *Fiscal year 1985: Study of runaways and youth*.

Yates, G., MacKenzie, R., Pennbridge, J., & Cohen, E. (1988). A risk profile comparison of runaway and non-runaway youth. *American Journal of Public Health, 78*, 820–821.

7 HIV Prevention for Youths in Independent Living Programs: Expanding Life Options

Wendy F. Auslander, Vered Slonim-Nevo, Diane Elze, and Michael Sherraden

The incidence of human immunodeficiency virus (HIV) infection among adolescents is increasing. Youths who were abused and neglected and in out-of-home care are among those at highest risk of acquiring HIV. The concurrence of sexual activity and school failures contributes to their high-risk status. Research suggests that changing behaviors of troubled youths requires programs that not only include HIV-related knowledge, attitudes, and skills, but also incentives and skills for educational planning that will expand the future life options of these youths.

Wendy F. Auslander, Ph.D., is Associate Professor of Social Work, George Warren Brown School of Social Work, Washington University, St. Louis, MO. Vered Slonim-Nevo, D.S.W., is Senior Lecturer, Spitzer Department of Social Work, Ben-Gurion University of the Negev, Beer Sheva, Israel. Diane Elze, M.S.S.A., is Social Work Doctoral Student, and Michael Sherraden, Ph.D., is Benjamin E. Youngdahl Professor of Social Development and of Social Work, George Warren Brown School of Social Work, Washington University, St. Louis, MO.

Youths who are abused and neglected and in out-of-home care are among those at highest risk of acquiring HIV [D'Angelo et al. 1994]. The concurrence of sexual activity, family instability and disruption, behavioral and emotional problems, and school failures contributes to their high-risk status. Although cognitive-behavioral strategies appear promising, they have had limited success in maintaining long-term behavioral changes. This article presents a conceptualization of HIV prevention for adolescents in independent living programs that links the reduction of HIV-risk behaviors with expansion of youths' life options through educational planning. Independent living programs, created by P.L. 99–272 and authorized by an amendment to Title IV-E of the Social Security Act, are funded under a federal entitlement and delivered by state child welfare agencies to prepare and support youths in their transition from out-of-home care to self-sufficiency and independence. HIV prevention should be an integral part of preparing youths for this transition and for survival.

This article presents (1) the characteristics of youths in the child welfare system that place them at risk of HIV infection; (2) previous attempts at HIV prevention used with this population, and their limitations; (3) data that provide a rationale for designing HIV prevention programs with a life options perspective; and (4) a strategy to prevent HIV infection that includes educational planning and the provision of assets for youths in out-of-home care.

Risk Characteristics of Youths in the Child Welfare System

Youths involved with the child welfare system usually present with psychosocial problems associated with risk behaviors that make them vulnerable to HIV infection. These problems include histories of physical or sexual abuse, neglect, family instability and disruption, poor health, educational deficits, substance abuse, and delinquent behaviors [Barth 1990]. One of the risk factors of adolescents leaving the out-of-home care system is limited educational options that diminish their life chances for economic and social stability [Cook 1994; DeWoody et al. 1993]. A national evaluation of independent living programs by Westat found that only 44% of 18-year-olds discharged from out-of-home care had completed high school [Cook 1994]. The study identified other educational deficits that included histories of grade retention, placements in special education, and disruptions in school attendance. Despite these problems, only 44% of the youths in the study received services in educational planning [DeWoody et al. 1993].

Youths in out-of-home care are also characterized by a high rate of pregnancy and sexually transmitted diseases. Forty-two percent of the youths surveyed in the Westat study reported giving birth to or fathering a child within one year of discharge [DeWoody et al. 1993]. Barth [1990] found that of youths discharged from out-of-home care for at least one year, 17% had a sexually transmitted disease and 40% reported a pregnancy. These data suggest that youths in out-of-home care are at risk for HIV infection because of their involvement in unprotected sexual activities. The combination of educational deficiencies and sexual risk-taking among these youths multiplies their risk for HIV infection. In fact, Slonim-Nevo et al. [1995] found that among youths in out-of-home care, educational deficits were positively associated with HIV-risk knowledge, attitudes, and behaviors.

Slonim-Nevo et al. [1991] found that troubled youths in residential facilities were highly knowledgeable about AIDS, but held few positive attitudes toward prevention and participated in unsafe HIV-related behaviors. Among runaway youths in shelters, substance use was found to increase vulnerability to HIV infection—investigators found that substance use was associated with having an increased number of sexual partners and with reduced frequency in condom use [Koopman et al. 1994]. Although runaway youths demonstrated high levels of AIDS knowledge and beliefs that supported AIDS prevention, only 18% reported consistent condom use [Rotheram-Borus & Koopman 1991]. Jemmott and Jemmott [1993] also found that urban youths who had sex while using alcohol and other drugs were more likely to engage in risky sexual behaviors such as sex with multiple partners and insertive anal intercourse.

Several studies have been conducted with youths in detention facilities. Nader et al. [1989] found that compared with public high school students, youths in a detention facility knew less about AIDS, perceived less personal threat of AIDS, felt less confident about preventing AIDS, and engaged in highly risky sexual activities. Gillmore et al. [1994] reported that delinquent youths in a detention facility were not consistently using condoms; condom use with casual partners was only 30%, and with steady partners only 16%. In addition, Gillmore et al. [1994] found that youths held negative attitudes about condoms; the youths believed that condoms reduced sexual pleasure, were artificial and unromantic, and interrupted sex. DiClemente et al. [1991] found that incarcerated youths, when compared with in-school youths, were less likely to know the protective value of condoms, initiated sex at an earlier age, reported more sexual partners, and seldom used condoms. Clearly, youths with multiple psychosocial risk factors, particularly educational deficits, limited future options, and sexual risk-taking behaviors require innovative HIV-prevention efforts that go beyond HIV risk-reduction practices. HIV-prevention programs must acknowledge the real obstacles faced by these youths in achieving independence and self-sufficiency.

HIV Prevention Efforts with Troubled Youths

Cognitive-behavioral interventions have been shown to be effective in the prevention of HIV transmission. In particular, Kelly and his colleagues developed a model of risk reduction that includes HIV risk education, cognitive-behavioral self-management training, and sexual assertion training that was successfully implemented with gay men [Kelly 1995; Kelly et al. 1990]. Further support for a cognitive-behavioral approach comes from other studies in which skills-oriented interventions changed HIV-risk behaviors among adolescent substance abusers [Marcus & Swisher 1993], minority youths [St. Lawrence et al. 1995], and troubled youths [Auslander et al. 1992; Rotheram-Borus et al. 1991; St. Lawrence et al. 1994]. The main assumption of the cognitive behavioral approach is that individuals engage in high-risk activities not because they lack relevant information, but because they lack the behavioral and cognitive skills necessary to use available information [Bandura 1977; Kelly 1995]. Thus, if youths acquire skills such as planning, problem-solving, decision making, and assertive communication, the desired change will be achieved.

Several efforts have been made to prevent HIV or reduce HIV risk behaviors through cognitive-behavioral skills training among troubled adolescents at risk. In the only controlled study of HIV prevention with youths in out-of-home care, the effectiveness of a skills-training program was evaluated in relation to reducing HIV risk behaviors, changing attitudes, and increasing knowledge of HIV prevention [Slonim-Nevo et al. 1996]. The skills-training program comprised nine sessions delivered over a three-week period, with each session lasting 1.5 to 2 hours. Youths who received the intervention were divided into small groups of approximately 8 to 10 youths per group. The program was delivered by master's level social work students who participated in 40 hours of HIV prevention training. Program content and the group leader training protocol are detailed elsewhere (see Slonim-Nevo et al. [1993]).

The short-term impact of the intervention was evaluated by comparing pre- and postintervention scores on HIV-related knowledge, attitudes, behavioral intentions, and behaviors [Auslander 1993; Auslander et al. 1992]. Youths in the treatment condition reported higher knowledge about HIV [$F(2, 264) = 11.75$, $p < .0001$], safer attitudes [$F(2, 260) = 9.81$, $p < .001$], and lower intentions to engage in HIV-risk behaviors [$F(2, 246) = 15.36$, $p < .0001$] than youths in the control condition. Of five risk behaviors assessed (males: vaginal sex without a condom, anal sex without a condom; females: vaginal sex without a condom, oral sex without a condom, anal sex without a condom), there was a significant decrease in females' reports of oral sex without a condom ($p < .05$) among youths in the experimental conditions when compared to those in the control group condition.

A second intervention study using a cognitive-behavioral approach was successful in increasing condom use and decreasing high-risk sexual behaviors among runaway youths in a short-term (three to six months) follow-up evaluation [Rotheram-Borus et al. 1991]. Other studies have demonstrated positive outcomes after a short-term follow-up with youths who participated in cognitive-behavioral programs. Jemmott et al. [1992] reported fewer occasions of sexual intercourse, fewer sexual partners, greater use of condoms, and a lower incidence of anal intercourse among African American adolescent males at a three-month follow-up.

Although cognitive-behavioral approaches to HIV prevention appear promising for youths, controlled studies have shown that these interventions may not be successful in maintaining reductions in HIV-risk behaviors. In the previously described study [Slonim-Nevo et al. 1996] that followed youths for 9 to 12 months after the intervention, the cognitive-behavioral skills intervention failed to produce long-term reductions in the level of participation in high-risk behaviors among abused and neglected youths.

Educational Options and HIV Prevention

Research has provided evidence of a relationship between expanded life options (i.e., educational aspirations and successes) and HIV risk characteristics. Slonim-Nevo et al. [1995] found that educational aspirations and positive relationships with teachers significantly predicted AIDS-related knowledge, attitudes, and behaviors among 11- to 18-year-old youths in residential centers. Further analyses of those youths who were eligible for the independent living program (i.e., 244 youths in mid- to late adolescence) confirmed the previous results. After controlling for age, gender, race, and the agency from which each youth was referred, educational aspirations remained a highly significant predictor of the risk status of the youths. When sociodemographics were statistically controlled, teenagers who planned to attend college had greater HIV-related knowledge, held more desirable attitudes toward HIV prevention, and reported fewer intentions to engage in HIV-risk behaviors than teenagers who did not plan to attend college (see table 1). A logistic regression to identify the educational

TABLE 1
Unique Variance (Unique r^2) Associated with Educational and Sociodemographic Predictors of Knowledge, Attitudes, and Coping with High-Risk Situations (n = 244)

	HIV-Related Knowledge[1]	Attitudes for HIV Prevention[2]	Coping with High-Risk Situations[3]
Educational Performance	*Unique r^2*	*Unique r^2*	*Unique r^2*
GPA (1=A-C; 0=F or D)	ns	ns	ns
Failing in School (1=yes; 0=no)	ns	ns	ns
Skipping School (1=yes; 0=no)	ns	ns	ns
Fighting with Teachers (1=yes; 0=no)	ns	.02*	ns
Educational Aspirations (1=college; 0=no college)	.05***	.02*	.02*
Sociodemographics			
Sex	ns	ns	ns
Race	ns	.03**	.03***
Age	ns	ns	.02*
Agency	ns	.04**	.04**

Model Statistics:
[1] F (9, 234) = 2.61; $p < .01$; $R^2 = .09$
[2] F (2, 233) = 5.43; $p < .001$; $R^2 = .17$
[3] F (9, 226) = 6.74; $p < .001$; $R^2 = .21$
*$p \leq .05$, **$p \leq .01$, ***$p \leq .001$.

parameters that predicted engagement in HIV-risk behaviors (1=yes; 0=no) (see table 2) demonstrated that higher educational performance was associated with less risky sexual behaviors. Youths with higher educational aspirations were approximately a third as likely to use drugs with sex than youths with lower aspirations. Further, youths experiencing conflictual relationships with teachers were nearly three times as likely to engage in anal sex, more than twice as likely to engage in unprotected anal sex and sex with drugs, and four times as likely to trade sex for resources than were youths who did not fight with teachers.

TABLE 2

Results of Logistic Regression: Effect of Educational and Sociodemographic Predictors on HIV-Risk Behaviors (n=244)

	Odds Ratios					
	Anal Sex†	*Sex w/ Alcohol*	*Sex w/ Drugs*	*Trading Sex*	*Unprotected Vaginal Sex*	*Unprotected Anal Sex*
Educational Performance						
GPA	0.74	0.84	0.72	1.70	1.00	0.92
Failing in School	1.30	0.73	0.76	0.84	1.60	1.00
Skipping School	0.62	1.70	1.10	1.20	1.30	0.99
Fighting w/ Teachers	2.70**	1.70	2.30*	4.10***	1.40	2.40*
Educational Aspirations	1.50	0.71	0.38**	0.88	0.80	0.85
Sociodemographics						
Sex	1.20	0.69	0.70	0.77	1.20	1.6
Race	2.40**	0.61	0.21***	1.30	1.80	2.60**
Age	1.10	0.98	0.91	0.83	1.20	1.00
Agency	0.35*	0.24***	0.13***	0.25**	0.38*	0.42*
Model Statistics	χ^2=31.83***	χ^2=42.70***	χ^2=66.40***	χ^2=24.54***	χ^2=31.77***	χ^2=26.49**

*$p \leq .05$, **$p \leq .01$, ***$p \leq .001$

† In the chart, "anal sex" refers to ever having had anal sex. "Unprotected anal sex" refers to having had unprotected anal sex during the three months prior to entering residential care.

Programs that focus on changing knowledge, attitudes, and skills may not be sufficient to motivate youths to reduce their risky behaviors when they have few life options. Changing the behaviors of troubled youths requires programs that not only include HIV-related knowledge, attitudes, and skills, but also skills and incentives for educational planning that will expand their life options.

Life Options Theory and HIV Prevention Efforts

Life options theory provides a theoretical perspective that assists in understanding the challenge of maintaining safer sexual behaviors among adolescents in the child welfare system. Life options are opportunities provided by the social structure for an individual's social and economic advancement [Dahrendorf 1979]. According to Sherraden [1990, 1991], assets such as savings accounts or scholarships for education provide youths with expanded life options and produce psychological and social benefits (e.g., increased personal well-being, future orientation and aspirations, and personal efficacy and self-esteem). These life options, whether structurally limited or enhanced, are then internalized and shape individual behavior [Sherraden 1991]. Empirical evidence indicates that assets promote positive attitudinal and behavioral changes [Page-Adams & Sherraden 1997; Yadama & Sherraden 1996].

Youths who lack a belief that a high school education will make a positive difference in their future tend to drop out of school [Sherraden 1986]. Provided with assets that expand their life options, however, these youths may think and behave differently. Perceiving a concrete possibility for their future, they may act as if they have a future worth living. An integral part of disease prevention is believing that one's future is worth protecting. According to life options theory, when assets and expanded options are present, people begin to think about investing in, and planning for, their future.

Educational Savings Accounts for Expanding Youths'

Life Options

One strategy for expanding the life options of youths in out-of-home care is to link educational planning to HIV prevention programs. A way to increase educational options is to provide youths with educational savings accounts (ESA), specifically, funds they can use to pursue postsecondary education or vocational training. An ESA could be structured as a matched savings account, similar to an individual development account [Sherraden 1991], or as a fully funded account. An ESA would constitute an asset that would give disadvantaged adolescents a means to expand their life options if they were provided with the training and skills to use it effectively in their own behalf. For example, an ESA for postsecondary training could provide youths with some financial resources by which they could begin to plan realistically for their future education or job training. Creative solutions to the HIV problem among youths, such as ESAs, will of course demand creative fundraising strategies. Partnerships between child welfare agencies and private organizations such as foundations, local businesses, or academic institutions may offer avenues for developing ESAs for youths in out-of-home care.

Currently, ESAs have not been distributed to youths in the child welfare system; thus, their impact on changing youths' attitudes about their future, the completion of high school, and their vocational aspirations and achievements have not been evaluated. Other asset-based programs may indicate the potential of ESAs with youths in the child welfare system. For example, in 1980 Eugene Lang, a multimillionaire industrialist, promised college tuition to 61 sixth graders in Harlem. In an area with a 50% to 75% high school dropout rate at the time, almost all of those students graduated from high school and about 50% were enrolled in college by 1988. One plausible explanation for this program's success is that disadvantaged youths, when provided with life options and opportunities, began to think and behave differently. Lang's experiment has since grown into the "I Have a Dream" Foundation, which today provides educational opportunities to youths in many cities across the country.

Youths from more advantaged families may have access to assets in the form of home equity, savings accounts, and investments secured by parents and other relatives. Youths in out-of-home care, however, usually come from home environments in which they have experienced abuse, neglect, and deprivation. Many have experienced chronic instability from multiple placements. Seldom do youths in out-of-home care have the backing or commitment of a family or of family assets for their education and training. With increased life options through ESAs, youths may be more likely to perceive themselves as having a stake in the future. With educational goals and aspirations, youths will more likely protect themselves from HIV infection, pregnancy, and other events that could severely limit their opportunities and future well-being.

Conclusion

Current HIV prevention techniques with youths in the child welfare system have been ineffective in the long term [Slonim-Nevo et al. 1996]. HIV prevention efforts have been narrowly defined and usually limited to changing sexual behaviors. These efforts, though well-intentioned, have compartmentalized youths' sexual activities from the rest of their lives, as if their life experiences are not connected. HIV prevention efforts must be multidimensional in their approach to the lives of adolescents, particularly adolescents whose difficult circumstances may result in a lack of future orientation and educational aspirations and options. Those devising HIV prevention efforts must also acknowledge the substantial obstacles—especially educational deficits and limited financial assets—to safer behaviors that face these young people.

Independent living programs (ILPs) are ideal settings in which to deliver a broad approach to HIV prevention. ILPs are intended to prepare youths for a self-sufficient future, and HIV prevention skills overlap with other life skills. Currently, ILPs vary in the extent to which they deliver HIV-related information and skill building to participants; the content is often confined to group sessions on health and sexuality. HIV-related information and skills should be incorporated throughout the ILP curriculum, that is, into content on self-esteem, communication and decision-making skills, substance use, and educational planning. For example, ILP modules on increasing healthy coping skills can be modified to include HIV-risk situations (e.g., peer pressure to have sex) as examples of stressful life situations. The high rate of pregnancy among youths discharged from out-of-home care is evidence that these youths are also at a high risk for HIV infection. It is the responsibility of the child welfare system to provide systematic and comprehensive HIV prevention services for these youths.

In recognition of the influence of the social environment on behavioral change, adults significant to these youths must take the lead in reinforcing HIV prevention messages. For youths in out-of-home care, these adults may include their workers or foster parents, and/or the staff members of residential programs. State child welfare agencies must ensure that their staff members are adequately prepared to provide HIV risk reduction information and counseling to youths in out-of-home care. Providing educational savings accounts is a strategy that, when incorporated into ILP-sponsored HIV-prevention programs, may facilitate the development of an orientation toward the future. A future orientation, in turn, can motivate youths to protect themselves, their health, and their future. ◆

References

Auslander, W. F. (1993). The challenge of preventing HIV among troubled adolescents. *Prevention Forum, 13*(4), 12–17.

Auslander, W. F., Slonim-Nevo, V., Ozawa, M., Shepard, S., & Gehlert, S. (1992). *Comparison of skills training, discussion, and control groups to prevent AIDS among abused and delinquent youth*. Presentation at the Eighth International Conference on AIDS, July 19–24, Amsterdam, The Netherlands.

Bandura, A. (1977). *Social learning theory*. Englewood Cliffs, NJ: Prentice Hall.

Barth, R. P. (1990). On their own: The experiences of youth after foster care. *Child and Adolescent Social Work, 7*, 419–440.

Cook, R. J. (1994). Are we helping foster care youth prepare for their future? *Children and Youth Services Review, 16*, 213–229.

Dahrendorf, R. (1979). *Life chances: Approaches to social and .political theory*. Chicago: University of Chicago Press.

D'Angelo, L . J., Brown, K., English, A., Mein, K., & Remafedi, G. (1994). *HIV infection and AIDS in out-of-home care*. Washington, DC: Child Welfare League of America.

DiClemente, R. J., Lanier, M. M., Horan, P. F., & Lodico, M. (1991). Comparison of AIDS attitudes and behaviors among incarcerated adolescents and a public school sample in San Francisco. *American Journal of Public Health, 81*, 628–630.

Gillmore, M. R., Morrison, D. M., Lowery, C., & Baker, S. A. (1994). Beliefs about condoms and their association with intentions to use condoms among youths in detention. *Journal of Adolescent Health, 15*, 228–237.

Jemmott, J. B., & Jemmott, L. S. (1993). Alcohol and drug use during sexual activity predicting the HIV-risk related behaviors of inner-city black male adolescents. *Journal of Adolescent Research, 8*(1), 41–57.

Jemmott, J. B., Jemmott, L. S., & Fong, G. T. (1992). Reductions in HIV risk-associated behaviors among Black male adolescents: Effects of an AIDS prevention intervention. *American Journal of Public Health, 82*, 372–377.

Kelly, J. A. (1995). *Changing HIV-risk behavior: Practical strategies*. New York: Guilford Press.

Kelly, J. A., St. Lawrence, J. S., Betts, R. A., Brasfield, T. L., & Hood, H. V. (1990). A skills training group intervention model to assist persons in reducing risk behaviors for HIV infection. *AIDS Education and Prevention, 2*, 24–35.

Koopman, C., Rosario, M., & Rotheram-Borus, M. J. (1994). Alcohol and drug use and sexual behaviors placing runaways at risk for HIV infection. *Addictive Behaviors, 19*, 95–103.

Marcus, C. E., & Swisher, J. D. (1993). *Working with youth in high-risk environments: Experiences in prevention. CSAP Prevention Monograph 12*. Rockville, MD: Center for Substance Abuse Prevention(DHHS Publication No. SMA 93–2034).

Nader, P. R., Wexler, D. B., Patterson, T. L., McKusick, L., & Coates, T. (1989). Comparison of beliefs about AIDS among urban, suburban, incarcerated, and gay adolescents. *Journal of Adolescent Health Care, 10*, 413–418.

Page-Adams, D., & Sherraden, M. (1997). Asset building as a community revitalization strategy. *Social Work, 42*, 423–434.

Rotheram-Borus, M. J., & Koopman, C. (1991). Sexual risk behaviors, AIDS knowledge, and beliefs about AIDS among runaways. *American Journal of Public Health, 81*, 208–210.

Rotheram-Borus, M. J., Koopman, C., Haignere, C., & Davies, M. (1991). Reducing HIV sexual risk behaviors among runaway adolescents. *Journal of the American Medical Association, 266*, 1237–1241.

Sherraden, M. (1986). School dropouts in perspective. *Educational Forum, 51*(1), 15–31.

Sherraden, M. (1990). Stakeholding: Notes on a theory of welfare based on assets. *Social Service Review, 64*, 580–601.

Sherraden, M. (1991). *Assets and the poor: A new American welfare policy*. New York: M.E. Sharpe.

Slonim-Nevo, V., Auslander, W. F., Ozawa, M., & Gehlert, S. (1993). AIDS prevention for adolescents at-risk: Training social work students as leaders. *Journal of Teaching in Social Work, 7*, 89–106.

Slonim-Nevo, V., Auslander, W. F., & Ozawa, M. N. (1995). Educational options and AIDS-related behaviors among troubled adolescents. *Journal of Pediatric Psychology, 20*, 41–60.

Slonim-Nevo, V., Auslander, W. F., & Ozawa, M. N., & Jung, K. (1996). The long term impact of AIDS-preventive interventions for delinquent and abused adolescents. *Adolescence, 31*, 409–421.

Slonim-Nevo, V., Ozawa, M., & Auslander, W. F. (1991). Knowledge, attitudes and behaviors related to AIDS among youth in residential centers: Results from an exploratory study. *Journal of Adolescence, 14*, 17–33.

St. Lawrence, J. S., Brasfield, T. L., Jefferson, K. W., Alleyne, E., O'Bannon, R .E., & Shirley, A. (1995). Cognitive-behavioral intervention to reduce African American adolescents' risk for HIV infection. *Journal of Consulting and Clinical Psychology, 63*, 221–237.

St. Lawrence, J. S., Jefferson, K. W., Banks, P. G., Cline, T. R., Alleyne, E., & Brasfield, T. L. (1994). Cognitive-behavioral group intervention to assist substance dependent adolescents in lowering HIV infection risk. *AIDS Education and Prevention, 6*, 425–435.

Yadama, G., & Sherraden, M. (1996). Effects of assets on attitudes and behaviors: Advance test of a social policy proposal. *Social Work Research, 20*(1), 3–11. (Previously published as Working Paper 95–2, Center for Social Development, Washington University).

8 Shared Experiences: Three Programs Serving HIV-Positive Youths

Adam Tenner, Rudy Feudo, and Elizabeth R. Woods

This article presents the major components of three models of linked psychosocial care for HIV-positive youths and youths at high risk for HIV infection: YouthCare (Seattle, Washington), TOPS Program (Bridgeport, Connecticut), and Boston HAPPENS (Boston, Massachusetts). These models were developed to connect hard-to-reach and otherwise marginalized youths to needed services. All sites have successful programs that are well integrated with their communities' systems of care for HIV-positive adolescents. The projects share their program elements, successes, and challenges. Practical suggestions are offered to those interested in providing and evaluating youth-oriented HIV care programs.

Adam Tenner, B.A., is Project Director, YouthCare, Seattle, WA. Rudy Feudo, Ph.D., is Project Director, TOPS Program, Bridgeport, CT. Elizabeth R. Woods, M.D., M.P.H., is Project Director, Boston HAPPENS, Children's Hospital, Boston, MA. *This article is a collaborative effort by the three programs highlighted and is supported in part by Special Projects of National Significance (projects #BRH 970159–04–0, #BRH 970158–04–0, #BRH 970155–04–0) and by the Adolescent Health Training Program, Maternal and Child Health Bureau (project #MCJ-MA 259195), the Health Resource Service Administration, and the U.S. Department of Health and Human Services. This article's content is solely the responsibility of the authors and does not necessarily represent the*

In 1993, the Health Resource Service Administration's Special Projects of National Significance (SPNS) became the first federally funded adolescent HIV initiative. SPNS (Title V of the Ryan White Care Act) provided funding for 10 adolescent-focused grantees to design, implement, and evaluate model programs that serve the needs of HIV-infected adolescents and young people. Projects were invited to provide site-specific evaluations as well as to participate in a crosscutting evaluation of all ten grantees.

Several of these programs, while having different designs, share similar experiences and provide a range of programming for hard-to-reach youths (street-involved, homeless, inner-city, ethnic minorities, and sexual minorities). The projects described in this article include the Boston HIV Adolescent Provider and Peer Education Network for Services (HAPPENS) Program at Children's Hospital (Boston), YouthCare (Seattle), and the Teen Outreach and Primary Services (TOPS) Program (Bridgeport, CT). All of these agencies provide integrated continua of care services for HIV-positive young people and youths at risk for HIV infection. These services include outreach, case management, early intervention, medical services, and youth development programming, as well as linkages with other local youth and child welfare resources.

This article supplies practical information on how three diverse sites, in three different cities, created effective programs that serve youths with HIV and those at risk for HIV infection. These young people are often vulnerable, with past histories of abuse, neglect, and homelessness, and may be runaway or throwaway youths due to sexual identity issues. They are at increased risk for child welfare involvement, homelessness, and HIV infection. Information about individual programs and practical suggestions for providers of youth services and child welfare services wishing to set up similar programs are included. Crosscutting data from the 10 grant-

---

official views of the above organizations. The authors thank their program staff members, youths, network participants, and colleagues in the 10 Adolescent SPNS initiatives, the Measurement Group, and the HRSA/SPNS staff for their support and encouragement. For further information on the 10 SPNS grantees, contact the Measurement Group at 310/215-7061 or visit their web site at http://www.tmg-web.com.

ees have been collected for the last three years in conjunction with The Measurement Group (TMG).* The evaluation consists of service encounter information and in-depth psychosocial interviews with individual youths receiving case management services.

Literature Review

HIV appears to be increasing among youths and young adults at a higher rate than in the general population. In addition, adolescents represent one of the most medically underserved populations in the United States and a need for models of services has developed [Blum 1987]. It is known that infection with sexually transmitted diseases (STDs) may increase the risk of transmission of HIV as well as offer a marker of risk-taking behavior. Unfortunately, less than half of adolescents with histories of survival sex, injection drug use, same-sex behavior, or a sexually transmitted disease associated with genital ulcers or sores has sought or received help for these HIV-related behaviors [Stiffman & Earls 1990]. Adolescence is often a time of experimentation and heavy use of alcohol and other drugs, and this is especially true for youths who are separated from their families or are survivors of abuse. Use of alcohol and other recreational drugs contributes substantially to potential HIV exposure [Elifson et al. 1993; Edlin et al. 1994]. Alcohol and drugs impair judgment, increase the likelihood of teens' participating in risk-related sexual behavior, and reduce the likelihood of condom use [Friedman et al. in press; Hingson et al. 1990].

There are between half a million and two million homeless and runaway teenagers in the United States today [Ryan & Futterman 1997]. Many homeless youths have run away from family violence and sexual abuse [Ryan & Futterman 1997] or are throwaway youths because of sexuality issues. These adolescents may exchange sex for food, shelter, or drugs in order to survive (survival sex) [Friedman & Goodman 1992; Morey & Friedman 1993; Sondheimer 1992]. This population needs special attention by all health care providers and by trained outreach workers [Melchiono 1991; Fried-

* The Measurement Group is a health-related evaluation company that specializes in HIV-related programs.

man et al. 1990; Rawitscher et al. 1995; Sugarman et al. 1991; Rotheram-Borus et al. 1991b; Schor & Goodman, in press; Cauce et al. 1994]. Street youths are often alienated and disenfranchised from established institutions. Many have chronic health and nutritional problems including STDs, poor oral hygiene, alcohol and drug addiction, hepatitis and HIV infection; a history of physical and sexual abuse; and mental health problems, including an increased risk of suicide [Morey & Friedman 1993; Pfeifer & Oliver 1997; Kipke et al. 1997; Embry & Lohr 1996].

All three programs gained from the knowledge and experience of other programs for HIV-positive and homeless youths. The Adolescent AIDS Program at Montefiore Medical Center in New York City demonstrated the importance of outreach to referring agencies to connect youths to sources of care [Futterman et al. 1993; DiLorenzo et al. 1993]. The Los Angeles system of care for homeless youths demonstrated the importance of collaborating with agencies in a defined geographic area, solidified by frequent network functions, to care for homeless and street youths [Yates et al. 1991; Kipke et al. 1993; Kipke et al. 1995]. Larkin Street Youth Center in San Francisco established a central drop-in center and medical clinic for HIV-positive street youths [Goulart & Madover 1991]. The Centers for Disease Control and Prevention [1996] demonstrated the need for HIV interventions in specific communities to be "based on local needs" and the importance of using a theoretical framework to develop prevention. The Health Resource Service Administration has provided guidelines from the Ryan White Title I programs for evaluation of local HIV service delivery programs that emphasize the importance of using qualitative and quantitative methods to evaluate service provision, consumer opinions, and HIV-related outcome measures.

The Projects

Though the projects' program components vary slightly, all three have common elements: outreach, case management, adolescent-specific HIV test counseling, a wide referral network, youth involvement, and peer education. Each project began by collecting qualitative data through focus groups and interviews with youths and local area providers. The key to the success of all three projects has been the creation of networks of youth services and medical providers. Figure 1 shows the common elements as well as the site-specific elements of the three projects.

While YouthCare serves more street-involved and homeless youths than the other projects, all three projects serve youths who are marginalized from traditional resources (i.e., family, schools, support networks). Many of the youths are involved in the child welfare or juvenile justice system. Many also face the added pressures of racism, sexism, and homophobia. All three projects have made special efforts to connect with agencies serving gay, lesbian, bisexual, transgendered, and questioning youths. All of these youths are at high risk for HIV infection and do not fit the profile of traditional HIV-positive people seeking medical and social support. A description of youths served by the projects can be found in table 1.

Boston HAPPENS

The Boston HAPPENS Program provides high quality, accessible, youth-oriented, culturally sensitive care for HIV-positive, homeless, and at-risk youths. Familiar faces, welcoming confidential care settings, and facilitated transportation have helped to maintain youths in needed services. For HIV-positive, homeless, and at-risk youths, any impediments can become barriers to care. Meeting youths where and when they choose is necessary to connect these hard-to-reach populations to needed social and medical services.

The Boston HAPPENS Program is a collaboration of adolescent-specific medical, outreach, case management, HIV counseling, mental health, and public health providers from the entire Boston area. The program provides a range of services to connect HIV-positive, homeless, and at-risk youths to adolescent-specific primary care and makes referrals to HIV specialty care. A particular emphasis is placed on connecting homeless youths from the Combat Zone in the Boston Commons area to services.

The program offers outreach, access, and coordination of eight core agencies, nurse case management, mental health services and

FIGURE 1

Elements of the Models of Care

Common Program Elements

- Outreach
- Adolescent-specific HIV test counseling
- HIV-positive youth speakers
- Hiring of youths in staff roles (peer educator and peer counselor)
- Case management of HIV-positive youths
- Extensive networks of youths, HIV, and medical service providers
- Basic needs services (i.e., food, clothing, and shelter)

Program Specific Elements

Boston HAPPENS

- Peer outreach and risk-reduction counseling
- Mental health support
- Health status screening and needs assessment services
- Primary and referral care services
- Nurse case management
- Multidisciplinary team care
- Follow-up and outreach to ensure continuity of care
- Integrated care and communication among providers in the metropolitan Boston area

YouthCare, Seattle

- Street outreach
- Outreach at local needle exchange sites
- Local drop-in center coverage and linkage
- Case management services for HIV-positive youths and youths at high risk for HIV infection
- Support, social, and treatment education services by and for young people with HIV
- Access to drop-in, shelter, and crisis intervention services

TOPS, Bridgeport

- Confidential and anonymous HIV counseling and testing on site
- Street outreach
- Social networking
- Mental health support
- Peer counseling and education
- Recreational opportunities
- Risk-reduction activities

TABLE 1
Client/Consumer Profile

	Boston HAPPENS	YouthCare	TOPS
	n (%)	*n (%)*	*n (%)*
Ages Served	12–25 yrs. (98.0)	14–25 yrs. (100.0)	15–24 yrs. (100.0)
Out-of-age range	(2.0)		
Gender			
Male	543 (36.3)	464 (55.9)	1312 (57.0)
Female	902 (60.3)	363 (43.7)	902 (39.2)
Unknown		3 (0.4)	87 (3.8)
Ethnicity			
Caucasian	801 (53.6)	535 (64.5)	121 (5.3)
African American	303 (20.3)	48 (5.8)	1438 (62.5)
Native American		25 (3.0)	28 (1.2)
Latino	208 (13.9)	30 (3.6)	551 (24.0)
Asian/Pacific Islander	57 (30.8)	36 (4.3)	42 (1.8)
Multiethnic	50 (3.3)	122 (14.7)	
Unknown	55 (3.7)	34 (4.1)	27 (1.2)
Sexual Orientation			
Heterosexual	889 (61.5)	480 (57.8)	2019 (87.7)
Gay/Lesbian	46 (3.2)	185 (22.3)	38 (1.7)
Bisexual	25 (1.7)	115 (13.9)	57 (2.5)
Undecided/Unknown	10 (0.7)	61 (7.3)	101 (4.4)
Homeless/Runaway	195 (13.0)	373 (44.9)	83 (3.6)
HIV Positive			
Males	24 (57.0)	22 (73.0)	6 (50.0)
Females	18 (43.0)	8 (27.0)	6 (50.0)

*Note: Percentages are rounded and may not total 100%.

supervision, peer support, connection to mental health and substance abuse services, primary care, and specialty HIV and adolescent care. The eight core agencies include two multiservice outreach agencies situated on the Boston Commons, three Boston hospitals (two private and one public), and three community health centers, all of which provide adolescent-specific services. This coalition of agencies provides services to homeless youths, African American and Latino youths, and gay and lesbian youths. Based on the experiences in health care delivery in Boston and other cities, the Boston HAPPENS Program model provides a citywide network of culturally and developmentally appropriate adolescent-specific care [Kipke et al. 1995; Yates et al. 1991; Futterman et al. 1993; DiLorenzo et al. 1993; Goulart & Madover 1991; Sondheimer 1992; Morey & Friedman 1993].

In organizing the network of providers, an informal group of adolescent-specific providers met regularly prior to any funding. These meetings provided support for coordinated care for HIV-positive youths and for the development of an HIV care educational forum. When collaborative funding was found through Special Projects of National Significance, the establishment of a formal care network and an educational program, and the enhanced recruitment of providers and agencies serving HIV-positive youths, was possible. The program has developed an essential role in the identification and care of youths with HIV / AIDS in the metropolitan Boston area.

YouthCare

YouthCare was founded in 1974 as the first shelter for runaway and homeless youths in Seattle and was one of the first nationally funded shelters under the federal Runaway and Homeless Youth Act. YouthCare's services are diverse and represent both traditional child welfare concerns as well as programming specific to runaway and homeless youths. YouthCare provides a wide array of services to street-involved, homeless, and sexual minority youths including emergency shelter, transitional living, drop-in, and outreach. The program has established excellent working relationships with social service and medical providers around the Seattle area.

Through initial assessments of HIV services in Seattle-King County, YouthCare found that adolescent-specific HIV test counseling services and case management services for youths who tested HIV positive were not available in Seattle. YouthCare designed a program that would meet the many needs of HIV-positive youths as well as those of youths at high risk for HIV infection [Rotheram-Borus et al. 1991b]. The program was designed so that the staff members could provide the full range of services, including outreach, HIV counseling and testing, case management, and support services.

In the first year, the project director established working agreements and relationships with local clinics that were identified by youths in focus groups as recommended HIV testing sites. At the same time, the staff members created working relationships with both the local drop-in centers for street-involved, homeless, and sexual minority youths, and with the local needle exchange sites.

The early emphasis of the program on outreach and setting up the network of service sites gradually began to change after the first year. YouthCare began to accept referrals for HIV-positive clients from local AIDS service providers. Many of these agencies were not ready for the level of service needed by youths with histories of street-involvement, homelessness, and mental illness. In many cases, co-case management arrangements were created. The standard arrangement was for YouthCare to provide primary case management and for the AIDS Service Organization (ASO) to provide ancillary services, as long as the health care and insurance coordination needs were minimal. In cases where youths became medically disabled, or youths "aged out" of the program, the roles would switch.

Over the years, the case managers have struggled to find a balance between outreach and case management. Though it was first considered that case managers would have a maximum active caseload of 30, YouthCare now understands that a caseload of that size is impractical because HIV-positive youths require much more time and energy than other clients, especially during the early phases of case management. As experienced by all three projects, an enormous amount of time is required to keep young people engaged in the level of medical service demanded by HIV. Given the broad scope of work, a maximum active caseload of 15 youths has been instituted.

TOPS

At TOPS, a range of HIV health care services and prevention activities was established by the agency. A 25-agency Greater Bridgeport HIV/AIDS Care Consortium existed, but it was a loosely structured, weak, deliberative body, not decisive and not representative of the target population of minority, hard-to-reach street adolescents. Strategies for improving linkages with individual agencies and the AIDS Care Consortium were initiated to improve the quality of services and access to those HIV care services for the TOPS population.

The Teen Outreach and Primary Services (TOPS) model is based on, and built upon, the principles of community outreach, peer support, and social networking as developed and implemented by the Bridgeport Women's Project, funded by the National Institute on Drug Abuse (NIDA). From 1988 to 1992, this street-based program sought out female prostitutes and female partners of injection drug users through a number of community-based strategies. The women were recruited and enrolled in a range of interventions for reducing the risk for HIV-infection and AIDS. Using the lessons learned from the Women's Project, TOPS adapted similar strategies for reaching HIV-infected and HIV-affected adolescents: increased outreach and the expansion of access to primary and specialty health care and support services.

TOPS provides outreach and primary care health services by skilled, streetwise staff members who are ethnically and culturally sensitive and who understand the target population. A group of peer educators was recruited from the target population; they were trained, paired with staff members, and supported in providing outreach services. Services include HIV counseling and testing, street outreach, case management, social networking, peer education, mental health support, risk-reduction counseling, and recreational activities. TOPS's target population is HIV-positive youths and youths at risk for STD and HIV infection who traditionally do not use or who underutilize social, health, educational, and community resources due to sociocultural, ethnic, or economic obstacles. These youths often do not have full access to the range of health and supportive services that can prevent or reduce HIV infection or transmission. Many of the youths do not have adequate medical, financial, educational, and social resources.

History of Youth Involvement

The field of social and medical services has been moving toward including clients/consumers in the design, implementation, and evaluation of services. While most of this movement has happened in systems serving adults, there is a growing clamor to involve youths in those services that affect them and their lives. Youth involvement has been a common thread throughout these three projects. Youths have been involved in the early setup of the programs and have been incorporated as staff members in all three projects. While it is often difficult to train and supervise youths who have had no previous job experience or who are living in homeless shelters or in out-of-home care, the benefits of doing so greatly outweigh the costs. Involving and hiring youths in programs have three primary benefits.

1. Youth service agencies are equipped to understand the complexities involved in youths' lives and teach basic job skills. This training can include the importance of showing up on time, boundaries at work, communication, computer skills, and writing resumes.
2. Youths trained as peer educators often benefit the most from peer education programs. Being able to retain a job where youths feel they are giving back to their communities and helping others often increases self-efficacy and self-esteem.
3. Providing job skill training and employing young people offers yet another opportunity for agencies to give back to the larger communities in which they operate.

Boston HAPPENS

Youths have been involved in the development and functions of the Boston HAPPENS Program since its inception. A high school student joined the project in its first year to help design the youth components. Shortly thereafter, a Youth Advisory Board was formed and began developing a youth brochure as well as providing feedback to the program. Youths representing HIV-infected and HIV-affected youths, transgendered youths, and youths of color attended peer leadership training. Four of these peer leaders were hired as youth staff members for the program. They have been active in waiting room outreach at local medical sites and street outreach with the program's Outreach and Services Coordinator in the Downtown Crossing and Roxbury areas. The peer leaders have spoken and staffed Boston HAPPENS' tables at many community events and health jams (summer neighborhood health information programs for youths) and have written several articles for newsletters and public releases. They have also appeared on television and radio and have had input into the city government through the Mayor's Youth Advocacy Day and the Massachusetts HIV Prevention Planning Group. To incorporate youths' opinions and views into the model, several youth focus groups, involving 20 diverse youth representatives of the program population, were held. The main questions explored the youths' views of what was needed from ideal health care sites and providers. This effort gave youths a voice and resulted in valuable contributions to the initial development of the program. What was heard was that youths preferred providers who spoke their language, maintained confidentiality, and gave support on issues facing them. They preferred care at a neighborhood health center or ambulatory care teen clinic. Periodic reassessment by focus groups and consumer surveys has been extremely helpful in continuing to meet the needs of the youths served.

Boston HAPPENS has been so active, and its youth activities have been so extensive, that the program is developing a position for a Youth Coordinator to supervise these activities. The Youth Coordinator will train and supervise a new group of peer leaders. He or she will also develop a youth speakers' bureau and help prepare youths for, and escort them to their presentations. The Youth Coordinator will also supervise the dissemination of program information and activities to the various youth communities. In addition, the Youth Advisory Board was reinitiated with representatives from community health centers and local agencies. Youths' participation has been an essential component for the success of the program.

YouthCare

Throughout the course of the project, YouthCare has continually increased the level of youth involvement. The experience of other youth service sites such as Bay Area Young Positives and the Health Initiatives for Youths in San Francisco suggested that youths could play important roles in the development and implementation of programs. This approach was instructive in developing services in Seattle.

The original program design set out to establish a network of HIV testing sites that street youths could easily access. To accomplish this, youths were consulted in focus groups and interviewed on such topics as where they received health care; where they received information on HIV; how many sessions should be included in an HIV pretest; and where would be good places to have HIV testing. Youths identified local drop-in centers and free health clinics for homeless youths as the best places to provide testing. They also emphasized that test-counseling sessions should be as short as possible. When asked where they received information on HIV, youths cited parents, TV, school, drop-in centers, and individual counselors.

An Adult/Youth Advisory Group (AG) was established to help plan the direction for the project. The AG included YouthCare's Youth Peer Educators (two youths hired from the populations they served), Youth Peer Educators from the People of Color Against AIDS Network, staff members from the Northwest Family Center (a Ryan White Title IV program serving women and families with HIV), the Seattle-King County Department of Public Health, and Children's Hospital. The AG met every two months for the first year of the project.

As the number of HIV-positive clients involved in the project rose, several young people began to organize and ask for new programming. In 1995 and 1996, YouthCare was able to send youths to the meetings of the National Alliance of Positive Youths in Washington, D.C. These meetings of HIV-positive youths from around the country were an inspiration for the young people. One particular youth was motivated to start a support group by and for young people with HIV. Programming by other agencies (e.g., Metro Teen AIDS in Washington, D.C.) also inspired him. YouthCare looked to other models of service to refine the design of its program. All interested youths participated in designing the program of Seattle's Positive Youth (SPY) and are largely responsible for its success at reaching young people with HIV. SPY began as a support and social group for HIV-positive young people in 1996. A second social group for female clients was formed in 1997. Thus, YouthCare evolved its youth involvement from focus group input to a program run by and for HIV-positive youths.

TOPS

During the initial implementation phase of the TOPS model, the project recruited and trained young people as peer educators from the target population of minority, hard-to-reach street adolescents. These young people served as the bridge between the target population and the service delivery system and were matched with outreach and case management staff members who were selected for their street experience and ability to establish rapport and trust within the community. Together, the peer educators and the senior staff members formed a cohesive team to provide outreach and early intervention services in a nonthreatening, nonjudgmental manner. This innovative model provides support and guidance to the peer educators through structured exposure to the senior staff.

The TOPS project began with the recruitment of 25 potential youth outreach workers for intensive Peer Leadership Training. Recruitment included, but was not limited to, individuals who were diagnosed with HIV infection or those who were sensitive to the project's goal of HIV reduction in Bridgeport. Of the 25 youths that began the Peer Leadership Training, only six were initially used as Peer Educators. Selection of Peer Educators was based on a number of objective factors, including consistent attendance, participation in all training sessions, attendance and participation in six individual training sessions with an experienced outreach worker, and successful completion of competency-based training goals (i.e., knowledge, skill, performance).

A team of experienced professionals provided training for the youth staff members. All training sessions were also attended by key project staff and community representatives from the juvenile court staff, human services staff, and so on. The youths that were not selected were engaged as resource volunteers. In the event that a selected peer did not complete the project year, one of the resource volunteers was hired as a replacement. Maintaining a core group of six Peer Educators available to provide ongoing services has been the project's standard practice.

Evaluation

When these projects were originally funded, a dual approach to evaluation was designed. TMG of Los Angeles, California, was hired as the crosscutting evaluator. SPNS, TMG, and the projects wanted to develop and evaluate individual program while also establishing a record of similarities and differences among the 10 sites that could be used to design future programs. The project sites have been using four quantitative forms to collect data as well as a combination qualitative/quantitative interview with youths enrolled in case management services. At this writing, data from these instruments are still being analyzed. Preliminary reports are available through TMG or its web site.

The projects were also concerned with evaluating their own progress and identifying how they were working as models of care for HIV-positive young people. The three projects took different approaches to the site-specific evaluation. Both Boston HAPPENS and TOPS used an integrated model of quantitative and qualitative data collection. YouthCare used a completely quantitative data collection system for the first three years and then switched to a more qualitative approach in year four. A summary of the program evaluations are included in figure 2.

Boston HAPPENS

Collecting information documenting community-based services and clinical information in a uniform manner is a challenge. Boston HAPPENS' data collection has been approached from a variety of directions. Given the wide range of agencies involved in data collection, ensuring the confidentiality and security of shared data was essential. Since Boston HAPPENS' evaluation takes place at many sites, program staff members have to interact frequently with all the sites to establish trust and ensure consistent data collection. Boston HAPPENS collects a wide range of data, including an evaluation of service availability collected in structured and qualitative interviews with area providers, mental health screenings, clinical intake of youths in the program, and consumer satisfaction forms.

It has been the experience of Boston HAPPENS that confidential systems must be adjusted to the specific clinical flow and the providers at each site. Booster training is necessary as network staff members change and information gathered is fed back to each site. Boston HAPPENS used such encouragement methods as inclusion in abstracts and papers as well as yearly reimbursement (in food and taxi vouchers, train tokens, and educational materials with additional funding) to motivate network staff members. Communication must be continual and positive to maintain the momentum. Boston HAPPENS employs an evaluator who is able to give regular and meaningful feedback to the project and the local sites.

YouthCare

YouthCare's evaluation approach has evolved with the program. When YouthCare began this project, there were no local services that targeted adolescents and young adults with HIV. The case

FIGURE 2
Description of Evaluation

Project	***Description***
Boston HAPPENS	• Encounter data including youth's risk behaviors, services provided, and referrals recommended • Clinically relevant in-depth interviews with HIV-positive youths that examine health, mental health, and substance abuse status for incorporation into medical records • Yearly overall evaluation of the structure of the network • Interviews and questionnaires completed by providers • Qualitative methods used include focus groups, feedback from training provided to youths and professionals, and consumer satisfaction questionnaires
YouthCare	• Original evaluation strategy included two basic components: (1) Community surveys ($n = 300$) to measure the impact and diffusion of information and behavior change on the community of street-involved, homeless and sexual minority youths (2) Consumer satisfaction questionnaires that measured satisfaction with the HIV test counseling services received • Redesign of site-specific evaluation includes emphasis on qualitative data collected in semi-structured interviews with youths using services, youths not accessing services, YouthCare's Case Managers and Project Director, AIDS service organization personnel who refer clients to YouthCare, and AIDS service organization personnel who do not refer clients to YouthCare
TOPS	• Qualitative interviews with young people include collection of data on teens' knowledge, attitudes, and behaviors that place them at risk for HIV infection; information on factors that contribute to utilization of, and compliance with, health care services • Interviews also touch on teens' and providers' perceptions of health care, prevention, education, counseling, testing, and partner/family notification • Changes in perceptions of above services monitored over time • Other data collected include histories of experience with homelessness, sexual abuse, family violence, relationships with families, peers, gender, sex roles and power differences • Quantitative data collected include basic demographics, HIV serostatus, compliance with health regimens, and perceived obstacles to care • Profiles for the following categories are generated for the entire sample, separately for each ethnic group represented, separately for males and females, and for each gender-ethnic group

managers provided outreach services to increase awareness of the project and to promote HIV testing for youths. YouthCare initially used a consumer satisfaction survey to evaluate the HIV testing component and a quantitative street interview or "community survey" to determine the range of risk behaviors, knowledge of HIV transmission, and the perceived factors that protect them from HIV. Over time and as the number of referrals for HIV-positive youths began to grow, the program emphasis shifted toward the case management needs of youths in the program. While the initial evaluation methods yielded some information about behaviors, attitudes (condom use, frequency of risk behaviors, etc.), and awareness of HIV services, they did not really assess the case management portion of the program. In the fourth year of the grant, YouthCare redesigned its evaluation methodology to focus on qualitative data pertinent to the case management aspects of the program. The new evaluation strategy will examine both YouthCare's program and the system of referrals within the AIDS service community. It should be noted that in the first three years, YouthCare oversampled gay, lesbian, bisexual, and transgendered youths. HIV disease in Seattle is still endemic to men who have sex with men (MSM). It was the agency's goal to make sure that this population was well represented in the evaluation.

TOPS

The evaluation of the TOPS project includes both process and outcome assessments. In addition, both quantitative and qualitative data are collected. The importance of an evaluation research design that combines both qualitative and quantitative data collection has been clearly demonstrated. Research has illustrated how qualitative techniques such as ethnography can go beyond objective analytic description to include description and analysis of the knowledge and beliefs that generate and interpret behavior [Patton 1992; Akins & Bescher 1980].

As part of ongoing training and evaluation activities, project staff members maintain daily logs on all peer educator activity. These logs have identified aspects of skill development, behavior, and street outreach that are critical to continued training and to modification of program strategies and direction. TOPS is currently evaluating how staff members and peer educators perceive training and supervision, and what factors serve as supports or obstacles to their performance. HIV test counseling has been an area of major challenge to service provision and evaluation. To understand this challenge better, this service will be evaluated by comparing on-site with street-based confidential and anonymous counseling and testing. The provision of two strategies will permit comparison as well as insight into obstacles and strengths in these two approaches.

Lessons Learned in Serving Vulnerable Adolescents

Networking and Working Agreements Are Paramount

There is an inherent challenge in creating a system of care for a population not normally reached through traditional avenues. Agencies in our communities often compete for funding and recognition of their programs. Even in a city like Seattle, historically known for its interagency collaboration, early discussions about how to provide services to people with HIV who were not disabled were heated. Ultimately, all communities have to find a balance between the needs of their organizations and the needs of the populations they are trying to serve.

When creating coalitions and networks, it is important to understand the needs of the individual staff members, their clients, and their agencies. Each collaborating agency has a different set of needs to address. A collaborative network program can adapt to the needs of each agency while retaining the integrity of the whole system. Some agencies may want to enhance their adolescent-specific services while others may need HIV counseling and testing, case management, or referrals to HIV care. Boston HAPPENS' staff members interacted with each of their collaborative partners to identify the interests and the needs of site staff members and optimize participation in the program. Ongoing definition of relationships is required as the staff changes over time. A flexible and diplomatic approach is essential for an integrated care model.

While it might not be practical to change the whole HIV service system in a community, there are ways to begin to advocate for HIV-positive youths. For example, YouthCare's linkages with health clinics for homeless youths, where YouthCare provides the HIV test counseling and the clinic provides the phlebotomy services, are an efficient model for social service agencies that cannot afford the expense or the liability of doing blood draws. At the same time, partnering with social service agencies enables health clinics to offer psychosocial support services for their clients and on-site HIV test counseling that medical providers often do not have time to provide. Partnering with community clinics to provide phlebotomy services helps provide better services to youths in communities.

At times, formal agreements are warranted. Formal resource and referral arrangements have been established by the TOPS project with 20 local provider agencies. The staff also helped improve interagency collaboration by strengthening the local HIV/AIDS Care Consortium in greater Bridgeport. This improved relationship among HIV service providers has resulted in the development of adolescent-specific clinics that address the multifaceted needs of high-risk youths in the Bridgeport area. A strong basis for collaboration has to be worked out before agreements and arrangements such as collaborative funding, weekly case conferences, and participation in evaluation and needs assessments can become a reality. If the member agencies of a local consortium do not trust each other, or if the membership of the consortium does not reflect appropriate representation from the infected or affected populations, there will be little support for service coordination and networking.

Case Management for HIV-Positive Youths Takes Time

In conversations among the authors and others over the first four years of the project funding, one issue has remained on the table—identified as an important message for program planners, service providers, planning counsels and consortia, funders, and policymakers—case management with HIV-positive youths takes time. This is probably not a shocking statement for most readers, but it has been the experience of these three projects that even the most seasoned case manager struggles to find enough time to work effectively with HIV-positive youths, especially during the early stages of enrollment and relationship building. Adjusting care and treatment plans to the lives of disenfranchised youths takes considerable negotiation. Youths with HIV often have complex lives that are exacerbated by poverty, homelessness, abuse, and ongoing risk-taking behaviors. Anecdotal reports from case managers at Boston HAPPENS and the other two sites have found that an early investment of time helps to connect youths to care before medical complications of HIV develop.

YouthCare's preliminary findings indicated that case managers spend an average of three or four times longer with HIV-positive clients than with their HIV-negative counterparts. Qualitatively, during the initial weeks, case managers might spend between five and 10 hours per week with a client. YouthCare has attributed the intensity of services at this initial phase to the clients' high level of unmet needs. There has also been some discussion that trauma and abuse history may be triggered when a young person receives an HIV-positive test result. The need to walk a young person through adult systems of HIV health care (which might include conversations about medications, insurance, benefits, appointments, medical procedures, etc.) can also be an exhaustive process for the youths and time-consuming for the case managers. Case managers often spend time after each medical appointment to help youths discuss and digest all the information that was given by the medical or insurance practitioner. This gradually tapers off as time goes on and the level of crisis experienced by the youths decreases. All three projects have experienced success in keeping clients involved in their own health care services by a generous allotment of time up front.

TOPS found that given the time intensity of working with HIV-positive youths, one staff person could not perform outreach and case management simultaneously. Outreach is a crucial and highly labor-intensive activity. Similarly, case management for HIV-positive youths is extremely time intensive. TOPS believes that in order to address all of the complex needs of infected youths, staff members must be available or at least accessible by phone seven days a week. Case managers must have a good relationship with the youths' primary care provider in order to offer the youths the needed services immediately. The window of opportunity is brief. Once youths are in the system, a great effort is required to maintain them in care.

System Changes May Be Necessary

The system of HIV care in the United States developed in the early years of the epidemic. The systems were set up quickly by and for the first community to be hit—gay and bisexual adult men—to meet the immediate medical and psychosocial needs of this community. Current systems of HIV prevention and care services are based on these original services. Although prevention services and technologies have evolved into more targeted and individualized interventions, services for people with HIV have remained broadly defined. When confronted with a mainstream care system designed primarily for Caucasian adult gay men, disenfranchised youths quickly fall through the cracks. Services must reach young women and people of color (especially young gay and bisexual youths of color) who are increasingly caught up in the HIV epidemic. It is also important to note that many of the youths served in the three programs have been involved or should be involved in the child welfare system. This may require that state child welfare systems form task forces or working groups on HIV-related matters. Linkages to the criminal justice system are also necessary for coordinating care during and after incarceration.

Although care services have traditionally been prioritized for disabled individuals, many communities are now struggling with prioritizing services for people with HIV who are not disabled. Because many young people with HIV do not receive AIDS diagnoses until they are in their twenties or thirties, youths often have little or no access to food programs, housing, and drug assistance. These three projects have all worked in their local communities to make sure that youths have access to needed services as well as to the decision-making processes of Ryan White Planning Councils and Consortia.*

Youths must be cared for when and where they are willing and able to receive services. Because they often live outside of traditional family settings, disenfranchised youths often have not been taught the skills of making and keeping medical appointments. Sexual and ethnic minority populations may also have biases against trusting the traditional medical establishment.

HIV-positive youths frequently fall outside of traditional insurance coverage. Boston HAPPENS found that more than half of the youths requesting services had no coverage at all. Eligibility for Medicaid or Medicare for this population would be quite rare. Coordinated care, such as Boston HAPPENS, must cross traditional institutional impediments to provide access to services. Youths must be helped to negotiate these complex institutional and insurance systems if they are to successfully connect to care.

Community Norms Can Be Obstacles

HIV-positive youths frequently feel isolated from their communities. Disclosure to families, schools, employers, communities, or health care professionals is difficult. Many gay, lesbian, bisexual, and transgendered youths are thrown out of their homes and communities when their sexual orientations are disclosed. Youths of color may already feel discriminated against and isolated by racism. Recent immigrants may be struggling for acceptance in their communities. All of these difficulties are further complicated by the youth's HIV status. It is important to work with youths and their communities to strengthen support for HIV-positive youths and to optimize their quality of life. All three projects have worked

---

* Ryan White Planning Councils and Consortia are mandated community planning groups that prioritize funding for HIV services in large cities, regions and states.

hard to increase the visibility of, and services for, HIV-positive youths by maintaining a speakers' bureau, by placing case managers in community agencies, and by creating "safe and welcoming" spaces by and for HIV-positive youths.

Since 1993, YouthCare has seen a change in attitudes within the Seattle community toward HIV-positive young people. It is to the credit of the Seattle-King County community that it has made room at the table for HIV-positive youths. Even two years ago, many of the youths involved in the program had not disclosed their HIV status. For example, at Lambert House (the drop-in center for lesbian, gay, bisexual and transgendered youths) many of the youths did not feeling safe enough to disclose their status. This has changed, due in part to changes in media portrayals of HIV-positive people, staff members' attention to the issue, and to the increased awareness prompted by YouthCare's project.

Before the development of TOPS, there was little activity in Connecticut regarding adolescents and HIV. There was no system in place to provide intervention for youths with HIV/AIDS and those at risk for HIV infection. Three years after efforts to incorporate HIV adolescent-specific issues on the local and state levels began, a system is being developed and institutionalized to confront this important problem. Once the need for intervention for youths at risk for HIV was documented, those agencies that traditionally served youths were interested in incorporating HIV-related activities into their programs. Often, this means that the agency has accepted TOPS staff members to be co-located in their facilities. TOPS staff members and peer educators have also provided HIV-awareness trainings in those agencies. In addition, TOPS has been involved in the HIV planning consortia in Connecticut, acting as a voice for HIV-infected or HIV-affected youths. TOPS efforts in the last three years have changed the way service providers and planning bodies view HIV-infected or -affected youths.

Among the major obstacles to services targeting youths are the political and religious climates and local attitudes that make it difficult to provide effective HIV/AIDS education in the schools. TOPS has formed partnerships with local traditional service providers to provide culturally sensitive training for them. By doing this, TOPS brought about changes in some attitudes and norms, and heightened the perceptions of vulnerability to HIV among at-risk youths. TOPS also made AIDS education fun and lively, while maintaining confidentiality.

The managed care system does not work for all populations. Youth service providers often see firsthand the problems that youths face in accessing health care and support services. Many youth service providers referred youths to either the adult clinics or pediatric care for health care services. Youths need adolescent-specific clinics where staff members are knowledgeable about adolescent development and comfortable working with young people. HIV-positive youths face the added burden of a disease that requires special support and expertise in medical care management, and the services they need may not be available under managed care plans. Doctors who specialize in adolescent medicine may not have experience in the treatment of HIV/AIDS, while doctors who specialize in HIV and infectious diseases may not have training or experience in treating adolescents. This lack of experience may create a situation where the patient may not receive appropriate referrals to specialists or needed ancillary services. In addition, care for adolescents often assumes parental or guardian involvement in the child's health care needs and treatment. Street-involved and homeless youths are often disenfranchised from their parents and traditional family systems, and members of many ethnic and cultural minority groups may harbor a mistrust of medical systems.

The impact of managed care on marginalized populations such as HIV-positive youths is only just beginning to be apparent. It is incumbent on the projects serving HIV-positive and high-risk youths to advocate for youths with HIV before the projects enroll in managed care plans. In Bridgeport, the TOPS project became partners with a hospital HMO plan. The staff holds monthly case

FIGURE 3
Project Successes and Challenges

Boston Happens

Successes	*Challenges*
• Establishment of a formal linked care service network for HIV-positive adolescents • Community and agency outreach • Establishment of HIV counseling and testing services • Consistent providers who are visible at multiple sites	• Establishing the network of care across institutional hurdles • Social and economic issues faced by youths including insurance limitations, lack of free care, and unfamiliar environments • Communication across agencies and institutions • Increasing the capacity of the case management program.

Youth Care

Successes	*Challenges*
• Linkages with community clinics and drop-in centers • Adolescent-specific test counseling • Creation of a referral network of AIDS, youth, and medical service providers • Case management program • Preventive case management for youths most at risk for HIV infection.	• Adapting to the high level of service needs of HIV-positive youths • Meaningful youth involvement in program development, implementation, and evaluation • Attending to the needs of staff members • Keeping youths involved in services • Increasing caseload capacity as more young people request services.

TOPS

Successes	*Challenges*
• Establishment of a strong peer counseling component • Intensive street outreach • Individualized case management services • Linkages to medical care • On-site HIV test counseling services	• Refining peer counseling component • Achieving a balance between staff "street smarts" and "professional skills" • Creating linkages with TOPS' case management

conferences with the medical staff, case managers, substance abuse counselors, mental health specialists, and outreach specialists. A one-stop shopping approach is optimal, where many services that are requested by HIV-infected youths can be found on site. Figure 3 describes the programs' successes and challenges in implementing and evaluating the projects.

Discussion

These three models of care for HIV-positive youths and youths at risk for HIV infection offer examples for providers trying to establish similar programs. The models contain components of client, community, and agency outreach; case management; HIV testing and counseling; and coordination with health care services to reach populations that frequently do not access care even under the best of circumstances. Caring for these hard-to-reach populations is time intensive and calls for overcoming traditional institutional obstacles. Flexible collaborative agreements that evolve over time are necessary to link services. Case management and health systems should be adapted to meet the needs of disenfranchised youths. This means including youths in decision and planning processes as well as encouraging them to get involved in local Ryan White Planning Councils and Consortia. Program staff members must work with community and health care establishments to increase the system's awareness of the special needs of HIV-positive youths and to work toward reducing impediments to care.

Evaluation activities of models of care are essential to allow dissemination of lessons learned. It has been the experience of the three projects that a blending of qualitative and quantitative analysis provides the richest data on program successes and challenges. Again, the importance of involving youths in the process of evaluation cannot be stressed enough. Understanding the success and challenges of these three model programs will, it is hoped, assist others to develop networks of care for HIV-positive youths and youths at risk for HIV. ◆

References

Akins & Bescher. (1980). *Ethnography: A research tool for policy makers in the drug and alcohol fields.* Washington, DC: NIDA (DHHS Publication Number 80–946).

Blum, R. (1987). Contemporary threats to adolescent health in the United States. *Journal of the American Medical Association, 257,* 3390–3395.

Cauce, A., Morgan, C., Wagner, V., Moore, E., Sy, J., Wurzbacher, K., Weeden K., Tomlin, S., & Blanchard T. (1994). Effectiveness of intensive case management for homeless adolescents: Results of a 3-month follow-up. *Journal of Emotional and Behavioral Disorders, 2*, 219–227.

Centers for Disease Control. (1996). Community-level prevention of human immunodeficiency virus infection among high-risk populations: The AIDS community demonstration project. *Morbidity and Mortality Weekly Report Supplement, 45*, 1–24.

DiLorenzo, T., Abramo, D., Hein, K., Clare, G., Dell, R., & Shaffer, N. (1993). The evaluation of targeted outreach in an adolescent HIV / AIDS program. *Journal of Adolescent Health, 13*, 301–306.

Edlin, B., Irwin, K., & Farvoue, S. (1994). Intersecting epidemics—Crack cocaine use and HIV infection among inner-city young adults. *New England Journal of Medicine, 331*, 1422–1427.

Elifson, K., Boles J., & Sweat, M. (1993). Risk factors associated with HIV infection among male prostitutes. *American Journal of Public Health, 83*(1), 79–83.

Embry, L., & Lohr, Y. (1996). *Characteristics and mental health of homeless adolescents: Age and gender differences*. Seattle, WA: YouthCare.

Friedman, L., & Goodman, E. (1992). Adolescents at risk for HIV infection, AIDS and HIV infection in office practice. *Primary Care, 19*, 171–190.

Friedman, L., Johnson, B., & Brett, A. (1990). Evaluation of substance abusing adolescents by primary care physicians. *Journal of Adolescent Health, 11*, 227–230.

Friedman, L., Stunin, L. & Hingson, R. (in press). A survey of attitudes, beliefs, behaviors and knowledge about AIDS and HIV testing by adolescents and young adults enrolled in alcohol and drug treatment. *Journal of Adolescent Health.*

Futterman, D., Hein, K., Reuben, N., Dell, R., & Shaffer, N. (1993). Human immunodeficiency virus-infected adolescents: The first 50 patients in a New York City program. *Pediatrics, 91*, 730–735.

Goulart, M., & S. Madover. (1991). An AIDS prevention program for homeless youths. *Journal of Adolescent Health Care, 12*, 573–595.

Hingson, R., Strunin L., & Berlin, B. (1990). Beliefs about AIDS, use of alcohol and drugs, and unprotected sex among Massachusetts adolescents. *American Journal of Public Health, 80*, 1–5.

Kipke, M., O'Connor, S., Palmer, R., & MacKenzie, R. (1995). Street youths in Los Angeles: Profile of a group at high risk for human immunodeficiency virus infection. *Archives of Pediatric and Adolescent Medicine, 149*, 513–519.

Kipke, M., Boyer, C., & Hein, K. (1993). An evaluation of an AIDS risk reduction education and skills training (ARREST) program. *Journal of Adolescent Health, 14*, 533–539.

Kipke, M., Simon, T., Montgomery, S., Unger, J., & Iversen, E. (1997). Homeless youths and their exposure to and involvement in violence while living on the streets. *Journal of Adolescent Health, 20*, 360–367.

Melchiono, M. (1991). Outreach to sexual minority street population, adolescents and youths. *Community Street Outreach Guide.* MADPH publication, 16 (547–63–1000–4–91 C.R).

Morey, M., & Friedman, L. (1993). Health care needs of homeless adolescents. *Current Opinion in Pediatrics, 5*, 395–399.

Patton. (1992). *Qualitative evaluation and research methods.* Beverly Hills, CA: Sage Publications, Inc.

Pfeifer, R., & Oliver, J. (1997). A study of HIV seroprevalence in a group of homeless youths in Hollywood, California. *Journal of Adolescent Health, 20*, 339–342.

Rawitscher, L., Saitz, R., & Friedman, L. (1995). Adolescent's preferences regarding human immunodeficiency virus (HIV)-related physician counseling and HIV testing. *Pediatrics, 96*, 52–58.

Rotheram-Borus, M., & Koopman, C. (1991a). Sexual risk behaviors, AIDS knowledge, and beliefs about AIDS among runaways. *American Journal of Public Health, 81*, 206–208.

Rotheram-Borus, M., Koopman C., & Ehrhardt, A. (1991b). *Homeless youths and HIV infection. American Psychologist, 46*, 1188–1197

Ryan, C., & Futterman, D. (1997). *Lesbian and gay youths: Care and counseling. State of the art reviews: Adolescent medicine*. Philadelphia: Hanley & Belfus, Inc.

Schor, E., & Goodman, E. (1998). Out-of-home living arrangements. In S. Friedman, K. Schonber, M. Fischer, & E. Alderman (Eds.), *Comprehensive Adolescent Health Care*. (pp. 718–722). St. Louis, MO: Mosby Year-Book, Inc.

Sondheimer, D. (1992). HIV infection and disease among homeless adolescents. In R. DiClemente (Ed.), *Adolescents and AIDS: A generation in jeopardy* (pp. 71–85). Newbury Park, CA: Sage Publications, Inc.

Stiffman, A., & Earls, F. (1990). Behavioral risks for human immunodeficiency virus infection in adolescent medical patients. *Pediatrics, 85*, 303–310

Sugarman, S., Hergenroeder, A., Chacko, M., & Parcel, G. (1991). Acquired immunodeficiency syndrome and adolescents. Knowledge, attitudes, and behaviors of runaway and homeless youths. *American Journal of Diseases of Childhood, 145*, 431–436.

Yates, G., MacKenzie, R., Pennbridge, J. & Swofford, A. (1991). A risk profile comparison of homeless youths involved in prostitution. *Journal of Adolescent Health, 12*, 555–560.

9 A Place Called HOPE: Group Psychotherapy for Adolescents of Parents with HIV/AIDS

Marianne Gunther, Sheila Crandles, Gillian Williams, and Margaret Swain

Project HOPE is a psychosocial support program for noninfected children of HIV-positive parents. The challenges of starting and implementing the program's psychotherapy group for grieving adolescents, and clinical examples of group process and effective interventions in group leadership, are described. Four stages in group development are explicated—safety, dependency, counterdependency, and independence—paralleling the adolescent separation-individuation process.

Marianne Gunther, M.P.S., is Program Coordinator; Sheila Crandles, M.S.W., is Program Supervisor; Gillian Williams, B.A., is Assistant Program Coordinator; and Margaret Swain, B.A., is Art Therapy Intern; State University of New York Health Science Center at Brooklyn, Brooklyn, NY.

As the end of the 20th century approaches, HIV is the number one cause of death for mothers of young children and adolescents. By the year 2000, over 80,000 children and adolescents nationwide will have been orphaned as a result of their parents' HIV disease [Michaels & Levine 1992]. The Report of the Working Committee on HIV, Children, and Families estimates that from 1981 through the end of 1996, 28,000 children and teenagers in New York State lost a parent to AIDS. By the end of 2001, the figure will be 58,000. These statistics represent not only the tragic loss of individual lives but also warn of a crisis in family and social responsibility [The Working Committee on HIV, Children, and Families 1996].

The HIV Center for Women and Children, based within the State University of New York Health Science Center, is located in central Brooklyn, an area with one of the highest incidences of HIV in New York City. It is estimated that Brooklyn will have 16,000 affected children and adolescents by the year 2001 [Levine 1993].

The need for support services for noninfected family members became evident to the Center's social work team when several mothers in a support group for infected women requested a separate support group for their noninfected adolescent children [Crandles et al. 1992]. In response, Project HOPE was established in 1991 and began offering confidential support groups for adolescent children, 12 to 17 years of age, who were aware of their parents' HIV serostatus. In 1995, the program expanded to include children nine to 11 years old. This article briefly describes the development of Project HOPE, highlighting the therapeutic benefits of the program's adolescent psychotherapy group. The four stages in the group's development parallel those in the adolescent's separation-individuation process. Clinical examples and a description of therapeutic interventions describe how the group ameliorates developmental disruptions from the trauma of parental illness and premature death. Also discussed are the unique challenges for professionals who work with this population.

Literature Review

The Impact of Death on Adolescents

The impact of the death of a parent during childhood has been extensively examined in the psychoanalytic literature [Bowlby 1981; Furman 1974; Wolfenstien 1966]. Bowlby found a correlation between early object loss and psychiatric depression. Wolfenstien found in many instances that the child, instead of detaching from the loved one and resolving the loss, has a greater attachment to the deceased parent and denies the finality of death.

Adolescents must mourn the various aspects of childhood that they are leaving behind as they move toward adulthood. During this developmental stage, they establish all kinds of personal limits. In confronting these limits, adolescents symbolically face mortality. If they are also challenged by contending with the actual death of someone they love, however, their coping capacities are stretched to the limits [Levy-Warren 1996].

For the adolescent who is losing a parent to AIDS, the grieving process is shrouded in stigmatization, secrecy, and shame. These individuals experience a double abandonment, one from the parent leaving them and one from a society that shuns them for being associated with AIDS. Negative attitudes concerning HIV/AIDS in both schools and the community can drive teenagers underground who are personally affected by HIV/AIDS [Draimin & McKelvy 1995].

In describing two time-limited support groups for children and adolescents whose parents have HIV/AIDS, Aaronson delineates the psychological crisis of these children:

> The loss of a parent is one of the most tragic and stressful events in a child's life. The connection between early object loss and psychopathology has been well documented in the literature. Children of HIV-infected parents are in a particularly unclear and difficult situation. They must

> maintain the precarious balance of continuing the normal routine of daily life while acknowledging that within several months or years, their parent could be lost to them forever. [Aaronson 1995: 223–235]

Adolescent Group Psychotherapy

Many adolescent therapists consider group psychotherapy to be the treatment modality of choice for adolescents. Scheidlinger [1994] attributes this to "adolescents' well-known hunger for peer group involvement." Adolescence is a time of rising psychosocial vulnerability where either psychopathology or self-actualizing can occur. Group therapy can provide the therapeutic environment wherein adolescents can work through interpersonal problems and examine the four basic identity questions: Who am I? With whom do I identify? What do I believe in? Where am I going? [Leader 1991].

Rachman has written extensively on group therapy with adolescents. He incorporates Erikson's developmental theory in his "identity group therapy model," whereby the group itself becomes the vehicle to assist adolescents with identity formation and consolidation [Rachman 1975]. Levin [1982] depicts the group as representing a transitional object that assists adolescents to individuate and separate from their families. Aaronson [1995] also promotes the benefits of group therapy and recommends further research and replication of this intervention with children of HIV-infected parents.

Project HOPE

Program Development

Project HOPE began in 1991 with the implementation of comprehensive adolescent psychosocial support services. Since that time, the program has continued to expand with the addition of two weekly therapeutic activity groups, a creative arts therapy group, and a homework group. In 1995, the program broadened the age range it encompassed to include preadolescent children 9 to 11 years old. Acknowledging the developmental differences of the two age groups, children ages 9 to 11 attend the homework and art therapy groups but do not attend the adolescent psychotherapy group. In addition to these support groups, individual and family therapy sessions are available for all age groups as needed. All activities and services take place in the State University's Student Center, which offers a friendly, youth-oriented, nonmedical atmosphere.

The goals of Project HOPE are (1) to assist youths with their anticipated loss and help them develop healthy coping mechanisms; (2) to diminish feelings of depression and shame secondary to HIV disease in the family and instill a sense of hope; (3) to lessen social isolation and foster an adolescent support network; and (4) to assist adolescents in successfully completing their separation and individuation tasks.

At this writing, Project HOPE has served 128 children between the ages of 9 and 18. The majority of the participants are from low-income, single-parent households with the mother as the primary caregiver. Eighty-five (67%) of the participants are African American, thirty-three (26%) are Latino, seven (5%) are from French or English Caribbean countries, and three (2%) are Caucasian. The ratio of males to females is 2:3. Seventy percent of the participants' parents have present or past histories of substance use.

Of the 128 children and adolescents in the program, 38 (30%) have experienced major separations from their parents and lived with other relatives or in family foster homes. To keep the family functioning, many of them have been cast in a parentified role and assumed the burden of adult responsibilities.

Referral Process

Program participants are referred by numerous sources, including inpatient and outpatient HIV medical services; HIV-related community-based organizations; out-of-home care, child welfare, and social service agencies; schools, and adolescent substance abuse treatment centers.

Radical change in the adolescent's behavior after a parent's disclosure of his or her HIV status is the most common reason for referral. The adolescent either acted out at home or at school, or withdrew from social activities and refused to talk to the parent about the illness. Other reasons for referral are parent initiated: the parent wants the child to be around other adolescents for support and wants a program to help educate the teenage child about HIV and AIDS.

Project HOPE works with the entire family and the intake interview is held with both the adolescent and parent. While the staff prefers face-to-face interviews, it is understood that the debilitating nature of the illness may prevent this. The program is therefore flexible about arranging interviews, conducting telephone interviews, meeting parents in the clinic, and on rare occasions, making home visits.

Parents wish to have their real concerns for their children acknowledged and supported. Very often the parents are anxiously expecting their own death and what this will mean for their adolescent child. As part of the interview process, staff members ask parents if they have planned for their child's guardianship and refer them to affiliated legal services. Staff members also encourage parents to seek support for themselves and recommend they consider joining an HIV support group offered at the site.

Children Living in Out-of-Home Care

A significant number of the children have been placed in family foster care or kinship care due to circumstances beyond their parents' illness. For example, one young girl lives in a family foster home because her mother was homeless and an active substance abuser. Another girl lives with her grandmother because her mother cannot afford an apartment large enough for herself and her children. In these circumstances, program staff members generally do not meet the biological parent, but work instead with the foster parent or guardian, as well as the case manager from the out-of-home care agency. Therefore, staff knowledge and understanding of the biological parent is solely based on what the child and guardians say.

Compared with adolescents living with their biological parents, teens in family foster care have a more urgent need to express their worries about their parents' health. Further, these teens tend to be strongly motivated to join the program and attend group sessions regularly. Very often the biological parent becomes idealized by the adolescent, who wishes for a reunion. At the same time, the guardian may want the adolescent to separate emotionally from the parent and move on. This causes much conflict between the teens and their guardians, because the guardians often resent the parent for getting infected, while the teen sees his or her parent as beyond reproach.

In working with these families, we found it helpful to take the time to talk to the guardian about the tremendous stress and conflict the adolescent is experiencing. The guardian often receives the brunt of the adolescent's displaced anger, causing the guardian to fight with the adolescent. Understanding and explaining this dynamic, validating the guardian's position, and offering a sympathetic ear are often all that is needed. We also recommend adult support groups for the guardians and encourage them to be aware of how all of this is affecting them. We encourage adolescents to discuss their conflicts in group and to explore their struggle in adapting to a new family while maintaining their loyalty to their parents.

Reasons Members Dropped Out

The death of a member's parent signifies the end of expecting grief and the beginning of the bereavement process for the adolescent. Members are encouraged to stay in the group for as long as needed. In general, adolescents at this stage of the bereavement process continue to attend group for about six months to one year.

Unfortunately, some group members have had to leave the group abruptly after the death of the parent, as they had to move in with relatives. Other reasons members leave are running away from home or being placed in out-of-home care, becoming pregnant and not returning after giving birth, travel to the program being considered too long, and becoming employed in an after-school job.

Leadership

Facilitating an adolescent group is often a difficult task. According to Scheidlinger, special knowledge, skill, and stamina are required of an adolescent group therapist to understand and deal with the intricate, "below-the-belly" kind of provocative testing and group-level resistance that characterize these groups, especially in the early phases. Further, he cautions that the adolescent group therapist "has to find a way to avoid being maneuvered into the role of the real parent, or other hated adults, or of behaving like "one of the gang" [Scheidlinger 1985: 102–111].

Leadership Styles and Functions

The program and assistant program coordinators of Project HOPE serve as coleaders of the group. Each leader brings her unique training, experience, and personal style to the group. In view of the prevalence of loss and death in the group population, group leaders place an emphasis on working with and strengthening relationships within the group. Encouraging group members to make attachments to each other, rather than to the leaders, helps them become more self-sufficient and less dependent on authority figures. Teenagers expecting the death of their parents tend to regress in their development, transferring their dependency needs onto the group leaders as the "group parents."

All group psychotherapy leaders must spend time educating group members on how to use the group in a therapeutic way; with adolescents, this is especially necessary. Members who have no understanding of the therapeutic group process will interact with each other as they would in any other social interaction. As with any new skill, leaders must guide participants, step-by-step, teaching them how to use the group to gain insight into themselves and their relationships with others. Simple ground rules should be established in the very beginning and members should agree on what behaviors will be tolerated. Confidentiality is a central concern for this population and is always the first rule members agree upon. Arriving and beginning the group on time and attending regularly are also essential. Last, and most important, members are expected to participate in the group process. To help members understand their value to the entire group, the metaphor of a basketball team is used. Teenagers quickly understand that the "game can't be played" if team members are missing.

Leaders must teach participants appropriate ways of communicating within the group. Given adolescents' tendency to be preoccupied with themselves, members tend to talk at the same time, cut each other off, and not listen to each other. They often direct their attention to the leaders as if they were in individual therapy. Group leaders then invite other members to respond, rather than responding themselves, to generate group discussion. Leaders demonstrate a curiosity and genuine desire to understand the feelings and experiences of each group member [Crandles et al. 1992]. The group leader's primary therapeutic role is to be a consistent and nonjudgmental container for all the intense feelings and questions these teenagers express in group sessions.

Coleadership generates a natural tendency on the part of members to try to divide the leaders. To avoid this, leaders must agree upon any policies or rules for the group and communicate regularly with each other about group behavior. Successful coleadership can be achieved when both group leaders meet weekly with a supervising group therapist to process the events and interventions of each group session.

Cultural Differences

Group leaders must constantly be aware of the cultural differences between members and between members and leaders, and encourage the group to discuss these differences. Many of the members have fixed beliefs about different ethnic groups. Since the members represent a mix of African American, Carribean American, and Latino cultures, many of these misconceptions surface in group discussion. The participants tend to be judgmental toward anyone who is different from themselves. Though adolescents typically insist on group conformity, the insistence seems especially strong for this group, who struggle with being stigmatized by their parents' illness. Leaders encourage members to discuss differences honestly and with respect, using these opportunities to learn about each other. Given the heightened awareness of differences, group leaders are aware of how their own cultural identities become part of the group dynamic.

Transference and Countertransference

In all forms of psychotherapy, it is natural for patients or clients to transfer onto the therapist or group leader their suppressed beliefs about, or wishes for, good parents. With adolescents—especially adolescents who are expecting the loss of their parents—this is especially true. Though they may deny or ward off feelings of dependency, most adolescents yearn for a compassionate adult to replace the parent they have lost. It is vital that professionals be aware of their countertransference responses to make sure they do not enact them. The wish to rescue the teen and become her or his parent is a common reaction. Weekly supervision with an experienced group therapist, regular discussions with one's coleader, and use of one's own psychotherapy are some of the methods used by the leaders to maintain awareness of their own countertransference.

Group Composition and Development

Presently, Project HOPE's psychotherapy group, known as Teen Talk, has 17 members. Ten core members regularly attend weekly group sessions (at least twice per month) while the remaining seven members attend less consistently (once every two months). In the past five years, over 100 adolescents have participated in Teen Talk.

With the shifts in membership, the group has experienced numerous cycles of group formation. Multiple hospitalizations of parents, the need to care for younger siblings, extracurricular school activities, and after-school jobs are among the most common stressors that cause teens to attend sporadically.

At this writing, in the fifth year of the program, members have endured a series of changes and losses within the group. One leader of Teen Talk who had been in the group for four years resigned, and several core group members left the group, leaving three remaining members. Two of these group members have been in the group for three years, while the third has been in the group for one year. These three group members have witnessed the deaths of several comembers' parents. One original member lost his mother the previous year and is just beginning to talk about her absence and his life without her. The group is getting to know the new coleader and to develop a relationship with her. Older members tend to direct their questions and needs to the senior group leader. New members do not have this transference element and are generally more concerned with feeling accepted and figuring out what will be expected from them, and what they can expect from the group. Subgrouping and competition for peer leadership are taking place, with two core female members tending to monopolize group discussion. A recurring theme for this group is the understandable and often internalized fear of being ostracized by peers.

Everyone is at a different level in his or her grief process. Some new members are in the early stage of denial and refuse to discuss their parent's illness, while other new members are eager to meet teens with infected parents and share their fears and feelings about their parents' health. While anger is often a palpable emotion in group sessions, many new members seem compelled to protect their parents from their angry feelings and deny feeling angry at their parents. They tend to displace this anger onto the leaders, or onto external forces such as the virus, society, or the medical community. Several participants have shared their magical belief that their anger could cause their parents to get sick and even die. Still others seem to have developed a false hope, as their parents continue to live through multiple hospitalizations, that their parents will defeat the virus and live forever.

In general, all group members become uncomfortable when periods of silence occur in the flow of group discussion, as if silence equals death. They often frantically try to fill up the space with trivial chatter. Leaders understand this manic behavior as a defense against facing the reality of their tragic situation.

Stages of Group Development

Gartner [1995] defines the group as a system that moves in levels of differentiation, from undifferentiated to differentiated. Initially, the group begins with no interrelationships—it is an aggregate of people, a roomful of strangers. As the group matures, relationships deepen and individuals become interdependent. Everything they do affects each other. Gartner describes four key stages in this differentiation process: (1) safety, (2) dependency, (3) counterdependency, and (4) independence. These stages are not linear; the group moves back and forth between them.

The stages of group development parallel the adolescent's separation-individuation process. For the group members, this process is thwarted by the threat of losing a parent. Although many teenagers are observed struggling to individuate, many others seem to share a merged identity with their ill parents. This latter group appears to feel responsible for their parents' happiness and well-being, which in turn can create guilt for desiring to separate and be autonomous. By encouraging members to experience autonomy within the group, leaders found that members were able to acknowledge their grief and begin to recognize their identity apart from that of their parents.

Stage 1: The Safety Stage

Adolescents are often reluctant to attend the group for various reasons. Teens tend to be suspicious of anything highly recommended by their parents. They can also have a tremendous fear that entering a therapy group means they are crazy, and that the group leaders will interrogate them or try to tell them what to do. Many members are frightened that they will encounter someone they know in the group and thus inadvertently disclose their parents' status to others.

The group began to reestablish itself approximately six months ago. The inconsistent attendance, attrition of old members, and addition of new members to the group impeded the ability of the group's members to build trust. Anxiety was heightened for new members who had no previous experience with group counseling or psychotherapy. In essence, the group was beginning again. At this stage of the group, members were figuring out what behaviors were acceptable or unacceptable, what would humiliate them, and what would help them feel comfortable. Members were recognizing similarities and differences in each other and seeking the commonality between them. Members from the previous group formation mourned the old sessions, saying how much easier it was to get a conversation going in the old group. These earlier members were not at first aware of the influence and powerful position they held in the pecking order of the group hierarchy [Gartner 1995].

In one group, members seemed to be experiencing the "hot potato" syndrome, in which they felt much anxiety about having the focus on themselves. Communication became a kind of game to get the attention away from oneself. An aura of politeness seemed to permeate the space, as members deferred to group leaders and hesitated to express their feelings. Leaders' efforts to engage members by asking questions were perceived as intrusive and interrogative. When one member described the sensation as "being on the hot seat," it was the turning point for the group, as the image helped members express their resistance and anxiety about having the focus on them. As members expressed irritation and frustration with the leaders for being "nosy," one group leader reminded the experienced members that the best way to limit the leaders' questions was for members to choose their own topics and begin group discussions. This gave the members a sense of control and empowerment.

Due to the stigmatization associated with HIV/AIDS, members tend to continually revisit the "safety" stage and initially want to deny the reason they joined the group. Common behaviors that indicate the need for safety are changing the subject, avoiding self-disclosure, discussing television talk shows or anything outside of the group, relentless teasing, and verbal fighting with each other or with the group leaders. In this way, the group members avoid authentic communication about themselves and their situation.

Stage 2: The Dependency Stage

In this stage, members take a dependent position, believing the group leaders will "cure" them [Gartner 1995]. The overall atmosphere is one of passivity. The group is continuing to work out aspects of safety and trust. Members are frightened of taking the initiative to start a group discussion and tend to sit back and wait for the leaders to intervene.

In one particular example, the leaders encountered a covert form of dependency in which scapegoating was used to avoid any real discussion. The group began with members who were at a loss for what to talk about and looking to the leaders to initiate discussion. The leaders suggested they review last week's group. This got the ball rolling but members had great difficulty staying focused on one topic and were easily distracted. Their conversation was tangential and evasive. Four influential members, who tended to scapegoat and monopolize, attempted to take over control of the group. When the group was interrupted twice by two members arriving late, these four members expressed their annoyance through their facial expressions, yet did not say anything. The other members would have ignored or avoided this conflict if the leaders had not pointed it out. The group leaders asked the group how they felt about the late arrivals and reminded them that they had been deciding as a group what the policy would be. At first, the members backed off from making any judgments, but as the leaders reemphasized that it was their group and their responsibility to create the rules, several members asserted the importance of being on time. Others shared how annoying it was to have to fill the late members in. The group decided it was up to the late members to ask questions and find out what was being discussed in the group. Then Vicki, a strong core member with much influence in the group, confronted Marie, who is quiet, about her silence. Vicki's complaints were supported by Nicole, an active and long-time member. The group became polarized between members who could not tolerate Marie's silence and members who empathized with her and felt she should not be pressured to talk. Initially the leaders encouraged members to talk to Marie rather than about her, thinking this might help her open up. As Marie continued to say nothing, Vicki and Nicole became increasingly hostile and aggressive toward her, even threatening to kick her out of the group. To reduce the scapegoating, the group leaders challenged Vicki and Nicole, saying that while they were pointing the finger at Marie for not talking and revealing herself in the group, no others in this session talked about their feelings or what was going on in their lives. In fact, Nicole's mother had recently been hospitalized and Nicole had not mentioned this to the group. Further, the leaders also wondered if someone could be different in the group and still have a place in it. While Vicki and Nicole seemed assertive by attacking Marie, they were actually still dependent on the leaders to steer and direct the group. Rather than talk about themselves or possibly challenge the leaders, the members displaced their aggression onto a passive member while also successfully filling the group session's time.

Stage Three: The Counterdependency Stage

In the counterdependency stage of development, group members are still dependent on the leaders but are fighting their dependency needs. Substantial conflict with those in authority characterizes this stage.

The group is presently in this developmental stage. Members are rebelling against the leaders and are externalizing their conflicts with authority. In a recent session, Tanya, a new member who attends sporadically, became extremely hostile toward Jose, when Jose shared his observation that several group members became quiet or turned in their seats whenever the topic of HIV or AIDS was raised. Tanya became extremely defensive, asking him if he was talking about her. She angrily said that she had turned in her seat because she had other things on her mind and found the group boring. She insisted that the topic of AIDS did not upset her. One leader gently reflected to her how angry she sounded, and she turned toward this leader and began yelling at her, saying she was angry with this leader for always picking on her and putting her on the spot. The group became extremely silent. As the leader believed that this was a good opportunity to open up and understand group members' anger, she asked if others felt the same way as Tanya did. Several members then criticized this leader's style. They complained that she asked too many questions. Others expressed frustration with the leader for not immediately understanding some of their expressions. Nicole said that she felt this leader was too "white" and therefore could not understand her because she was "black." Group members then explored the significance of race and language. Jose confronted the other leader, who is Carribean American, asking her why she was not "more like us" since she too was a person of color. Several members then began asking this leader where she was from and why she spoke differently than they spoke. Both leaders responded to the assault of criticisms and questions with self-restraint and tolerance. The Carribean American leader explored why the members thought she had to talk a certain way, just because of her race. The Caucasian leader acknowledged her difference and then explained that the reason behind her asking questions in the group was that she did not want to assume she knew what they were feeling and what their lives were like. When the tension subsided, the leaders acknowledged Tanya's anger and the complaints of others but wondered if the intensity of this anger was really meant for someone else, another adult in their lives who asked too many questions or put them on the spot. In this way, the explosive moment became an opportunity to help members understand the notion of transference, that is, of projecting their feelings about their parents onto the leaders. At the end of the session, Tanya apologized to Jose for yelling at him and admitted she was very upset and worried about her mother in the hospital.

The counterdependency stage can be extremely challenging for the leaders, making them feel intimidated and inadequate. If the group leader keeps in mind, however, that the anger and rebelliousness characteristic of this stage is not a personal attack, she or he will be in a better position to endure this phase. It is during the counterdependency stage that the group leader can most clearly observe and appreciate the emotional turmoil of the adolescent's separation-individuation process.

Stage Four: The Independent Stage

When a group reaches this stage, members have achieved autonomy [Gartner 1995]. They now have a sense of who they are and how they can continue in their lives. At this stage, the group's work is completed. While Teen Talk is not at this stage, there have been sessions in which the group has clearly made strides toward autonomy and individuation. Soon after the session described above, Jose came in and announced that the members would be choosing the topics for discussion. He then stated that Tanya had a topic she wanted to discuss. Tanya revealed that she was under tremendous stress in her home because of conflicts with her stepfather. She also revealed that she had recurrent thoughts about suicide. Several group members empathized with her and revealed their difficulties with their families and those times when they had considered suicide. In fact, two members had recently been hospitalized for suicidal gestures and they described their painful ordeal. As they discussed their suicidal feelings, members realized they really did not want to die, but wanted the pain to stop.

Unlike the previous session, where the members' anger at their parents was projected onto the leaders, in this session the members were able to talk about these powerful feelings openly with one another. As members were feeling very close to each other, the group had difficulty ending the session but agreed that the discussion would continue next week.

As members begin to differentiate from each other and assert their autonomy, they can reveal their feelings of sadness, anger, and despair. Before this session, members' energies were spent defending and protecting themselves. As members felt safer and increasingly less dependent on the leaders, they were better able to express their grief and bereavement. To help adolescents expecting the loss of their parents, they must deal simultaneously with their need to individuate. The group has (1) helped with anticipatory mourning; (2) lessened members' feelings of depression and shame and instilled hope for the future; (3) reduced isolation and helped create a social support network; and (4) helped adolescents separate psychologically from their parents in the prospect of their parents' terminal illness.

Summary

Working with any adolescent is a challenging task. The challenge is even greater when trying to help teens who are expecting the death of their parent. The following guidelines are helpful in working with HIV-affected adolescents.

Program Development

- Be flexible with parents during the intake process, i.e., arrange interviews in the most convenient manner possible for the family.
- When possible, hold program activities in a comfortable, pleasant, nonmedical setting.
- Engage adolescents in the therapeutic process by arranging nonthreatening, nurturing activities such as "pizza parties" to encourage trust.
- Provide adolescents with transportation reimbursement and snacks to encourage program attendance and retention.

Clinical Issues

- Decrease the intensity of group members' transference to the leaders as parents by making group rather than individual interpretations.
- Encourage group members to develop friendships among themselves. This often increases group cohesion and encourages self-sufficiency and independence from authority figures.
- Leaders must be aware of their own countertransference reactions to group members and process their feelings in weekly supervision sessions.

Adolescent Bereavement

- Professionals working with HIV-affected adolescents must recognize that members of this population may have extreme difficulty in making and keeping attachments in all aspects of their lives.
- Aggression is a normal part of the bereavement process for adolescents. As demonstrated in the group vignette in this article, outbursts must not be taken personally by the therapist. If the therapist can maintain neutrality and contain the aggression, some steps can be made to help the adolescents begin to understand their anger and find constructive ways to express it .
- There is no proper way to mourn the loss of a parent, especially for an adolescent. Adolescents should be allowed to grieve in their own way. For example, some teens may appear to be unaffected by their parent's diagnosis or death and may want to resume normal activities. This does not mean that they have no feelings about the loss.
- New guardians may need help understanding the adolescent's need to idealize their infected parent as a natural way to hold onto the parent and diminish the

stigmatization they may feel in being the child of an HIV-positive parent.

This article has described how group therapy parallels the individuation-separation process of adolescents whose parents are HIV-infected. The authors urge that programs incorporating group therapy be developed to meet the growing mental health needs of youngsters in this situation. ◆

References

Aaronson, S. (1994). Group intervention with children of parents with AIDS. *Group, 18,* 133–139.

Aaronson, S. (1995). Five girls in search of a group: A group experience for adolescents of parents with AIDS. *International Journal of Group Psychotherapy, 45,* 223–235.

Bowlby, J. (1981). *Attachment and loss. Volume III: Loss*. New York: Basic Books.

Crandles, S., Sussman, A., Berthaud, M., & Sunderland, A. (1992). Development of a weekly support group for caregivers of children with HIV disease. *AIDS Care, 4,* 339–351.

Draimin, B., & McKelvy, L. (1995). AIDS, adolescents, and bereavement: An overview. *The Networker, The Newsletter of the AIDS and Adolescents Network of New York, 6,* 2–10.

Furman, E. (1974). *A child's parent dies: Studies in childhood bereavement*. New Haven, CT: Yale University Press.

Gartner, D. (1995, March). *Stages of group development*. Unpublished paper presented at the State University of New York-Health Science Center at Brooklyn, Brooklyn, NY.

Leader, E. (1991). Why adolescent group therapy? *Journal of Child and Adolescent Group Therapy, 1,* 81–93.

Levin, S. (1982). The adolescent group as transitional object. *International Journal of Group Psychotherapy, 32,* 217–232.

Levine, C. (1993) *A death in the family: Orphans of the HIV epidemic*. New York: United Hospital Fund.

Levy-Warren, M. (1996). *The adolescent journey*. Northvale, NJ: Jason Aronson Inc.

Michaels, D., & Levine, C. (1992) Estimates of the number of motherless youth orphaned by AIDS in the United States. *The Journal of the American Medical Association, 288,* 3456–3461.

Rachman, A.W. (1975). *Identity group therapy with adolescents.* Springfield, IL: Charles C. Thomas.

Scheidlinger, S. (1985). Group treatment of adolescents: An overview. *American Journal of Orthopsychiatry, 55,* 102–111.

Scheidlinger, S. (1994). An overview of nine decades of group psychotherapy. *Hospital and Community Psychiatry, 43,* 217–225.

The Working Committee on HIV, Children, and Families. (1996). *Families in crisis: Report of the Working Committee on HIV, Children, and Families.* New York: Federation of Protestant Welfare Agencies, Inc.

Wolfenstien, M. (1966). How is mourning possible? *Psychoanalytic Study of the Child, 21,* 93–123.